Surgery in London

and

The Royal College of Surgeons of England

Opportunities and Pitfalls

John S. Bolwell

Grosvenor House
Publishing Limited

This book is published by
Grosvenor House Publishing Ltd
Link House
140 The Broadway, Tolworth, Surrey, KT6 7HT.
www.grosvenorhousepublishing.co.uk

A CIP record for this book
is available from the British Library

ISBN 978-1-80381-158-1
eBook ISBN 978-1-80381-159-8

CONTENTS

List of Illustrations

Tables

Introduction

The Royal College of Surgeons of England (RCS England) evolved directly from craft guilds established by the fourteenth century in the City of London. In 1796, the Company of Surgeons relocated to the south side of Lincoln's Inn Fields, Holborn where RCS England's extended but outdated 'Barry' building was completely rebuilt behind the façade and library between 2017 and 2021 at a cost of £79.7 million (See Fig. 1). Its neighbour to the east, the Nuffield College of Surgical Sciences (See Fig. 2), was built by RCS England to provide accommodation for 100 postgraduate students and opened in 1957. The London School of Economics (LSE), a constituent college of the University of London,

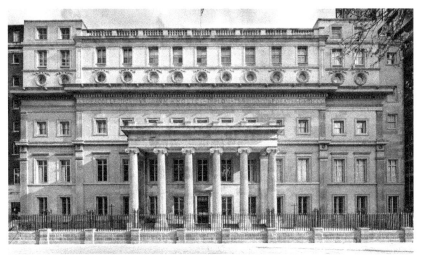

Figure 1. The Royal College of Surgeons of England, 39-43 Lincoln's Inn Fields, photograph 30 April 2021. The college was completely rebuilt behind the 'Barry' façade and library between 2017 and 2021.
Hawkins/Brown, architects.
Courtesy of fotohaus ltd.

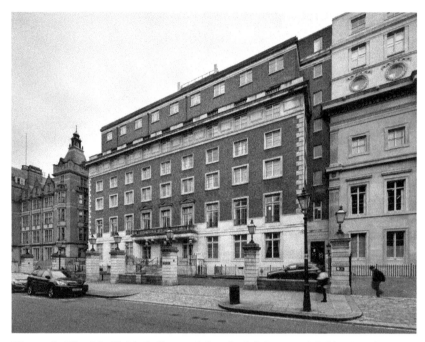

Figure 2. The Nuffield College of Surgical Sciences. 35-38 Lincoln's Inn Fields, completed in 1957 and acquired by the London School of Economics (LSE) in 2017, photograph 11 November 2021. The old Land Registry building, Nos. 32-34, purchased by the LSE in 2010 is seen to the east (left).
Alner W. Hall, MC, FRIBA, architect.
Courtesy of fotohaus ltd.

purchased a 155-year lease of the Nuffield building for £51.5 million in late 2017.

The old Land Registry building had been acquired by the LSE for £37.7 million and the Imperial Cancer Research Fund's Laboratories (See Fig. 3) for around £75 million in 2010 and 2013, respectively. Thus, the LSE, founded in 1895 by Fabian Society members Sidney and Beatrice Webb, Graham Wallas and George Bernard Shaw, became the owner of almost the entire south side of Lincoln's Inn Fields which, formerly, had been the

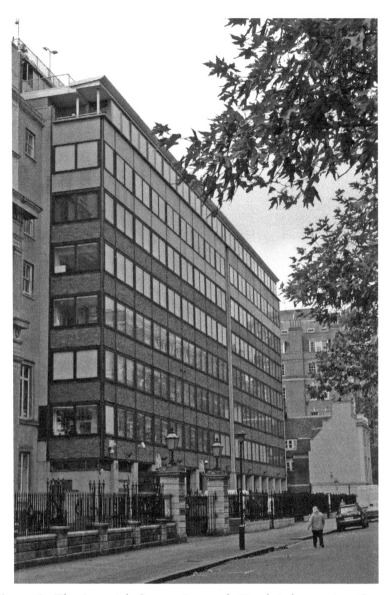

Figure 3. The Imperial Cancer Research Fund Laboratories (Cancer Research UK from 2002), 44-46 Lincoln's Inn Fields abutting RCS England, completed in 1963 , photograph 2008. It was acquired by the London School of Economics in 2013 and demolished in 2018.
Young and Hall, architects.
Courtesy of Cancer Research UK / Wikimedia Commons.

stamping ground of surgeons, surgeons-in-training and medical scientists.

The responsibilities of RCS England unexpectedly decreased after the Second World War during an era which was probably the most revolutionary in surgical history. Extraordinary advances were made in the medical sciences, engineering and high technology along with the groundbreaking techniques of minimally invasive surgery. The outcome was a dramatic expansion of the spectrum of disease amenable to surgical treatment.

The Royal Commission on Medical Education (the Todd Report) in 1968 proposed that undergraduate and postgraduate institutions should become an integral part of multi-faculty colleges of universities. London was considered separately because of the disproportionate number of historic teaching hospitals, medical schools, specialist tertiary referral hospitals and research institutes. The analogous recommendations of the Todd Report and the Flowers Report in 1980 for the University of London were still being negotiated in 1993 when Kenneth Calman, Chief Medical Officer for England, was commissioned by the government to replace the old United Kingdom (UK) system of specialist training in order to comply with European Union (EU) directives on 'harmonisation.'

The consequences for RCS England of Todd, Flowers and Calman included the demise of the Institute of Basic Medical Sciences, the Nuffield College of Surgical Sciences, Examination Hall, Down House, the Buckston Browne Surgical Research Farm and historic diplomas. In 2010, responsibility for surgical training was transferred to the General Medical Council and managed by Health Education England from 2012.

The only definitive history of RCS England was written by Sir Zachary Cope, MD, MS, FRCS (1881-1974) and published in 1959.[1] The archives of the college contained voluminous records most of which Sir Zachary perused with the assistance of Librarian, William Le Fanu (1904-1995) and Curator of the Hunterian Museum, Jessie Dobson (1906-1984) who, subsequently, became archivist to the Worshipful Company of Barbers. Decisions of Council were minuted but deliberations were secret so it was necessary to refer to contemporaneous medical journals to 'fully understand the questions at issue.' Sir Zachary was well-known to the profession as a member of Council and Vice-President of the college and also because of his useful and enjoyable book, *'The Acute Abdomen in Rhyme'* published in 1947 under the pen name 'Zeta.'[2]

A beautifully illustrated coffee table encomium entitled, *'The Royal College of Surgeons of England: 200 Years of History at the Millennium'* edited by Professors John Blandy (1927-2009) and John Lumley (born 1936) both former members of Council was published, without citations, in the year 2000. The book was intended to entertain and not to be relied upon as a secondary source.[3]

An account of the abovementioned transformation in medical education, surgical training and practice after the Second World War is presented along with details of the commissioned reports and some of the most consequential innovations! An overview, currently lacking, of almost 700 years of recorded surgical history provides requisite historical context including the sometimes adversarial relationship of diplomates with RCS England and its predecessors.

The ongoing controversy regarding the organisation of operative and postoperative surgical care that is currently a hot topic at home and overseas is discussed. This is because there is an increasing number of elderly patients and others with significant comorbidities at high risk of complications and mortality following complex procedures performed locally. Superior outcomes appear to be achieved by high volume surgeons working in high volume, regional or national, tertiary referral centres which specialise in specific open, laparoscopic and robotically assisted procedures. 'Failure to rescue' patients with complications appears to be associated with smaller hospitals.

RCS England invited Baroness Helena Kennedy, QC to produce a *'Diversity and Inclusion Review'* that was published on 18 March 2021. Sadly, it described widespread 'sexism, racism and homophobia' in the college and profession and called into question the organisational structure of RCS England. The college responded with a *'Diversity, Equity and Inclusion Action Plan'* (DEI) published on 16 September 2021 and the subject is reviewed.

The purpose of this mini-monograph is to provide a concise account of the evolution of surgical training and practice as it affected London and the rôle of the Royal College of Surgeons of England and its predecessors,

John S. Bolwell

References (Introduction)

1. V. Zachary Cope, *The History of The Royal College of Surgeons of England* (London: Blond, 1959), 360.

2. Zeta (V. Zachary Cope, author) and Peter Collingwood (illustrator), *The Acute Abdomen in Rhyme* (London: H K Lewis, 1947), 102

3. John P. Blandy and John S. P. Lumley, eds., *The Royal College of Surgeons of England: 200 Years of History at the Millennium* (London: Royal College of Surgeons of England; Oxford: Blackwell Science, 2000), 193

Acknowledgements

The author wishes to thank Saffron Mackay, Library & Archives Assistant, Susan Isaac, Information Services Manager and Rupert Williams, Director of Library and Archives: the Royal College of Surgeons of England; Pamela Forde, Archive Manager: the Royal College of Physicians of London; Peter Ross, Principal Librarian: the Guildhall Library (City of London), Inderbir Bhullar, Curator for Economics and Social Policy: Library of the London School of Economics; Sara Belingheri, Library Assistant and Amelia Walker, Senior Library Assistant: the Wellcome Collection; Tricia Lawton, Information Specialist: the Royal Institute of British Architects; Aisling O'Malley, Archivist: the Institution of Engineering and Technology; Victoria West, Archivist: the Worshipful Company of Barbers; Nicholas Wood, Honorary Curator and Past Master: the Worshipful Society of Apothecaries and Verus IT, Sydney, Australia for their contributions, suggestions and corrections, which have been gratefully incorporated into the manuscript.

Glossary

AES	Assigned Educational Supervisor's Report
ARCP	Annual Review of Competence Progression
Bart's	St. Bartholomew's Hospital, London
BBC	British Broadcasting Corporation
BMA	British Medical Association
CAT & CT	Computerised Axial Tomography
CCST	Certificate of Completion of Specialist Training
CCT	Certificate of Completion of Training
CST	Core Surgical Training
DEI	Diversity, Equality and Inclusion
DGCH	Deutsche Gesellschaft für Chirurgie (German Society of Surgery)
DM (Oxon)	Doctor of Medicine (Oxford)
DNA	Deoxyribonucleic Acid
DOPS	Direct Observation of Procedural Skills
ENT	Ear, Nose and Throat
EU	European Union
EWTD	European Working Time Directive
FFARCS	Fellow of the Faculty of Anaesthetists of 'RCS England'
FRCA	Fellow of the Royal College of Anaesthetists

FRCP	Fellow of the Royal College of Physicians of London
FRCS (Eng.)	Fellow of the Royal College of Surgeons of England (from 1843)
FRCS (Ed.)	Fellow of the Royal College of Surgeons of Edinburgh
FRCSI	Fellow of the Royal College of Surgeons in Ireland
FRCOG	Fellow of the Royal College of Obstetricians and Gynaecologists
FRIBA	Fellow of the Royal Institute of British Architects
FRS	Fellow of the Royal Society
GMC	General Medical Council
GOS	Hospital for Sick Children, Great Ormond Street, London
HEE	Health Education England
HM	Her or His Majesty
HST	Higher Surgical Training
ICL	Imperial College, London
ICSP	Intercollegiate Surgical Curriculum Programme
JCIE	Joint Committee on Intercollegiate Examinations
JSCFE	Joint Surgical Colleges' Fellowship Examinations
KCL	King's College, London
LC	Laparoscopic cholecystectomy
LDS	Licence in Dental Surgery, RCS England.
LETB	Local Education and Training Board
LRCP	Licentiate of the Royal College of Physicians of London

LSA	Licentiate of the Society of Apothecaries
LMSSA	Licentiate in Medicine and Surgery of the Society of Apothecaries
MB. BS	Bachelor of Medicine and Bachelor of Surgery
MCR	Multiple Consultants' Reports
MD	Doctor of Medicine
MFDS	Member of the Faculty of Dental Surgeons, RCS England
MMC	Modernising Medical Careers
MP	Member of Parliament
MRCS	Member of the Royal College of Surgeons in London (1800 to 1843)
MRCS (Eng.)	Member of the Royal College of Surgeons of England (from 1843)
MRCS (Ed.)	Member of the Royal College of Surgeons of Edinburgh
MRCSI	Member of the Royal College of Surgeons in Ireland
MRI	Magnetic Resonance Imaging
mRNA	Messenger Ribonucleic Acid
MS	Master of Surgery
MTAS	Medical Training Application Service
NHS	National Health Service
NMR	Nuclear Magnetic Resonance
OM	Order of Merit
OPHTH	Ophthalmology
ORL	Otorhinolaryngology

PBA	Procedure Based Assessment
PLAB	Professional and Linguistics Assessment Board
PRCP	President of the Royal College of Physicians of London
PRCS	President of the Royal College of Surgeons of England
PPRCP	Past President of the Royal College of Physicians of London
PPRCS	Past President of the Royal College of Surgeons of England
PPRIBA	Past President of the Royal Institute of British Architects
PRA	President of the Royal Academy
PRS	President of the Royal Society
PMETB	Postgraduate Medical Education and Training Board
QC	Queen's Counsel
QMUL	Queen Mary College, University of London
RA	Royal Academician
RCP	Royal College of Physicians of London
RCT	Randomised Controlled Trial
SGUL	St. George's Hospital Medical School, University of London
SHO	Senior House Officer
SI	Statutory Instrument
StR	Specialty Registrar (plus year of training e.g. 'StR3')

SpR	Specialist Registrar
SR	Senior Registrar
UCL	University College, London
UCLA	University of California Los Angeles
UCSF	University of California San Francisco
WBA	Work Based Assessment
WTR	Working Time Regulations

Addendum to Glossary

Pounds, Shillings and Pence

Prior to 15 February 1971, 'Decimal Day' in the UK, there were 12 pennies to the shilling and 20 shillings to the pound. There was a five pound note (fiver), a one pound note (quid), a 10 shilling note (10 bob, 10/-), a one shilling (1/- or bob - five shillings were called a dollar), half a crown (2/6 or half a dollar), a florin (2/-), a sixpence (tanner), a three penny bit (thrupenny bit or joey), a half penny (haypni) and a quarter penny (farthing). The old system, known as 'pounds, shillings and pence' dates back to Anglo-Saxon times (410-1066) when a pound of silver was divided into 240 pence, or denarii in Latin, which is the 'd' in 'Lsd' (librae, solidi, denarii) and was written, for example, as £1 2s. 3d. The £ sign is an elaborate 'L.'

A guinea contained a quarter of an ounce of gold mined in the Guinea region of West Africa and circulated between 1663 and 1816, Its value was fixed at £1 1s. 0d. in 1717 to prevent fluctuation with the price of gold. After 1816, the term guinea (and its value) survived as a unit of account used primarily for professional (medical and legal) billing and in horse racing, greyhound racing and the sale of rams! Gold sovereigns were last minted in 1603 and were struck again from 1817 but have not circulated in the UK since 1914. They are now bullion coins nominally worth one pound sterling.

I   Guilds in the City of London

Guilds (or Gilds) were founded in major towns and cities throughout Europe and the British Isles from the eleventh to the sixteenth centuries and formed an important part of the local economic and social fabric. In the City of London, the earliest charter still in existence was granted to the Weavers' Company in 1155. Guilds were an association of craftsmen or merchants formed for mutual aid and protection and for the furtherance of their economic and professional interests which included training by apprenticeship and the maintenance of high standards. There were 111 Guilds in the City of London's square mile by 1423 and there are 110 Livery Companies today that maintain only a tenuous connection with their original craft or trade. The word 'livery' refers to the uniform that identified each company.

Records preserved by the City of London and the Worshipful Company of Barbers confirm that a Company or Guild of Barbers and a Fellowship or Guild of Surgeon were in existence by 1308 and 1369 respectively and may have been established much earlier.[1] Members of the former were recognised as practitioners of surgery trained in the monasteries and more numerous than the latter who were primarily military surgeons with experience on the battlefield.[2] These two bodies evolved directly into the present day 'Royal College of Surgeons of England' (RCS England). There were similar craft associations in Bristol, Chester, Newcastle, Norwich and York modelled on London's Company of Barbers that was referred to as the 'Parent Company.' What is known about them was summarised by Sit John McNee (1887-1984) in a 'Thomas Vicary Lecture' delivered on 30 October 1958 at RCS England.[3]

In 1376, the Lord Mayor and Aldermen of the City of London issued ordinances to the Company of Barbers who had complained to the City about unskilled practitioners tarnishing its reputation.

The Ordinances provided for the inspection of surgical instruments and decreed 'that henceforth no man of their craft shall be admitted to the franchise of the said city if he be not attested as being good and able upon good examination before you made.'[4]

By the fourteenth century, aspiring members of craft guilds were required to undertake a seven-year, indentured apprenticeship to a master of their craft which was traditional at the time. According to Dobson and Walker (1979), new ordinances for the Fellowship of Surgeons were approved by the City of London in 1435. The 'usual rules' applying to 'the seven-year apprenticeship' were listed therein.[5] These ordinances were copied by a single scribe towards the end of the fifteenth century and bound in an 'Ordinance Book' which is preserved in the archives of the Worshipful Company of Barbers.[4]

In 1421, physicians trained in the earliest English and European universities were concerned that quackery was causing 'great harm and slaughter of many men' and presented a petition to Parliament.[6] This resulted in an order in the King's Council decreeing that those who had studied physic (physicians) must be licensed 'by their universities' and surgeons by 'masters of their art.'[6] The order was not enforced or followed by an Act of Parliament and had lapsed by 1423 along with an abortive attempt by the Faculty of Physicians and the Fellowship of Surgeons to form a 'Conjoint College of Physicians and Surgeons.'[6]

In 1462, the Barbers' Company was incorporated by royal charter granted by King Edward IV (r. 1461-1483) and officially became the Company of Barbers.[6] It was empowered to regulate the practice of surgery within a one mile radius of the City of London that was not extended to seven miles until 1629 by King Charles I (r. 1625-1649).[6] There was a 'composition' (but not an amalgamation) between the barbers and the surgeons in 1493.[6] A licence to practice surgery was issued, jointly, to Robert Anson on 8 August 1497 following his examination on 1 August 1497.[6] A copy of this licence (See Fig. 4), by the same scribe, is included in the aforementioned 'Ordinance Book.'[6]

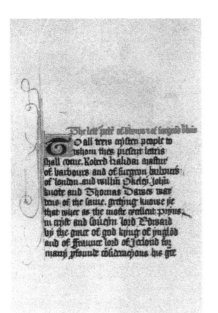

Page 1

Page 2

Page 3

Page 4

Figure 4. (*continued*)

Page 5

Figure 4. Copy of a five-page licence to practice surgery issued to Robert Anson on 8 August 1497, jointly, by the Company of Barbers and the Fellowship of Surgeons. The licence is written in Middle English and bound in the 'Ordinance Book' of the Fellowship of Surgeons. The book consists of copies made by a single scribe in the late fifteenth century. Courtesy of the Worshipful Company of Barbers.

**Figure 4. Transcription of Robert Anson's Licence to Practise Surgery, 8 August 1497
by R. Theodore Beck, 1974**

Page 1:   The letters patent of barbours and of surgeon barbours

TO all true Christian people to whom these present letters shall come, Robert Halidai master of barbers and of surgeon barbers of London and William Okeley, John Knots and Thomas Dawes wardens of the same greeting, know ye that whereas the most excellent prince in Christ and sovereign lord Edward by the Grace of God King of England and of France, lord of Ireland, for many profound considerations his grave

Page 2: moving, hath granted the well to him in Christ, the approved freemen the commonalty of barbers and of surgeon barbers of London, the search and oversight, correction and punishment, examination and approbation of all freemen using or haunting the cunning of surgery and barbery, and all manner of men foreigns using or haunting any particular part of surgery within the said city or suburbs thereof, as about new wounds old sores and other lesions whatsoever they be, also in drawing of teeth "ventosyng scarificacous" and such other manual operations like as the letters patent of our said liege lord the King thereupon made

Page 3: plainly may appear; we therefore the said Robert, William, John and Thomas at this time masters and wardens of the said Fellowship, for the common profit, wealth and relief succour of our lord the King's liege people, intending to provide men of good capacity and able in manners and cunning, sufficiently learned, informed and laboured by long experience, and other in the said craft of surgery; have prayed and required master John Smith doctor in physic, Instructor and examiner of the said Fellowship, and by the same for that intent chosen and elect to enter and examination for the causes above said, with divers persons which long time without authority, have used and haunted with experience the cunning

Page 4: of surgery whereupon after due and divers monitions made in this behalf, Robert Anson one of the said commonalty at the common hall of the same in London appeared, in his proper person, the first day of August last past, submitting himself to the examination and the apposition *[questioning]* where and when the said Robert by the said John Smith, in a great audience of many right well expert men in surgery and others, was openly examined in divers things concerning the practice operative and directive in the said craft of surgery. And there albeit he hath afore this many times been well approved, yet now he is newly abled by the said doctor and Fellowship, and

Page 5: found able and discreet to occupy and use the practise of surgery, as well about new wounds, as cancers, fistulas, vicerations and many other diseases and divers; and the same Robert thus approved and abled we have, as an expert man in the said faculty, approved and abled to occupy and practise in the said faculty, in every place, when and as oft as him best liketh we have licensed him and granted to him by these presents in witness whereof we have put the common seal of barbours and of surgeon barbers of London, given at London in the common hall of the said commonalty the VIII day of August the year of our lord God MCCCCLXXXXVII.

R. Theodore Beck. *The Cutting Edge: Early History of the Surgeons of London* (London: Lund Humphries, 1974): 149.

II   The Episcopal Licence and the Regulation of Surgery by Physicians

In 1511, an Act of Parliament authorised diocesan bishops (and the Dean of St. Paul's) to issue licences to physicians and surgeons after taking advice from 'expert persons in the said faculties.'[7] The 'freedom' of the Company of Barbers was required for episcopal licensure to practise surgery in London.[8] The established church in England was the *'Ecclesia Catholica'* under the primacy of the Bishop of Rome whose familiar title of Pope *(Papa)* is an unofficial one!

The first Act of Supremacy was passed in 1534 at the behest of King Henry VIII (r. 1509-1547) and marked the beginning of the English reformation. The King became the 'Supreme Head of the Church of England' and the clergy was obliged to swear an oath of allegiance.[8] The reformist Archbishop of Canterbury and Primate of All England, Thomas Cranmer (1489-1556), became the first Protestant to hold the office and acted on behalf of the King.[7] Cranmer was responsible for one of the glories of the English language, the *'Book of Common Prayer,'* that was published in 1549 in the reign of Edward VI (r. 1547-1553), son of Henry and Jane Seymour. Cranmer's nemesis was the Catholic Queen, Mary I (r.1553-1558), Henry's daughter by his first wife Catherine of Aragon, who had him burned at the stake!

There was a hiatus in the issue of episcopal licences between 1642 and 1660 during the Civil Wars and the Interregnum.[7] The practice was resumed after King Charles II (r. 1660-1685) was restored to the throne but 'gradually faded away' over the next century although the Act was not repealed until 1948.[7]

The College of Physicians was created by royal charter granted by King Henry VIII in 1518 and began to refer to itself as the Royal College of Physicians of London (RCP) after the Restoration in 1660.[6] University graduates became licentiates of the college

(LRCP after 1660) by passing an examination and paying an annual fee.[6] Graduation from the Universities of Oxford or Cambridge was required for election to the fellowship of the college (FRCP) and this bye-law, not abrogated until 1835, led to frequent protests and even rioting on one occasion in 1767 by non-Oxbridge licentiates.[6]

A second charter, in 1523, extended the powers of the RCP to regulate the practice of medicine and surgery from London to the whole of England.[2] Thus, the scene was set for almost 300 years of disputes with the barbers, surgeons and other medical bodies such as the Society of Apothecaries.[2] Some were consequential and had to be settled by Act of Parliament or the appellate jurisdiction of the House of Lords.[2] Surgeons were not university graduates and learned their craft by apprenticeship so were unable to assume the title 'Doctor.'[2] This led to the practice of entitling English surgeons, 'Mr. Mrs. or Miss,' that the surgeons chose to continue to this day.

III   The Worshipful Company of Barbers and Surgeons
1540 to 1745

In 1540, an Act of Parliament formed the 'Worshipful Company of Barbers and Surgeons' without a hyphen![6] The Act stipulated a sharp division between them; the only shared activity was the pulling of teeth.[6] The system of surgical apprenticeship, examination, eligibility for episcopal licensure and practice became the responsibility of the surgeon members only. The seven-year, indentured surgical apprenticeship was permitted in London from the age of 14 but, by 1743, a binding fee of between £100 (£25,591 in today's money)[9] and £250 (£63,977)[9] was required.[10] In addition, a candidate had to 'pass an examination in Latin.'[11] The apprentice was provided with board and lodging by the master usually in his own household. The consideration paid to a master barber in 1743 was £10 (£2,559)[9] and it is recorded that there were 'eighty-four bindings to barbers and five to surgeons' in that year![10]

At the conclusion of the indenture, the candidate underwent a *viva voce* examination by the Court of Examiners. If successful, he became a 'freeman' (or 'yeoman') to practise his craft. In the course of time, he became a 'liveryman' entitled to wear a uniform, participate in the election of the Lord Mayor and the two Sheriffs and take part in the City of London's ceremonial functions.[12] The title of 'sheriff' (or 'shire reeve') is of Anglo-Saxon origin (410-1066). The 'reeve' was the king's representative in a city, town, or shire (county) who was responsible for collecting taxes and enforcing the law. The liverymen constituted the 'electorate' and were eligible to be appointed, by seniority, to the 30 member Court of Assistants (15 barbers and 15 surgeons) and the 10 member Court of Examiners.[12] Members of both Courts were appointed for life! The Company was governed by four masters (two barbers and two surgeons) chosen annually and the principal master was alternately a barber or a surgeon also on an annual basis.[12] Those who accepted (or declined) the appointments paid a 'considerable fine,' or 'fee' in modern parlance.[1]

IV   The Company of Surgeons 1745 to 1800; John Hunter (1728-1793)

By the early eighteenth century, despite the persistence of the Hippocratic/Galenic 'school of medicine' that survived into the late nineteenth century, surgeons were becoming more skilled and numerous, not least. because of the voluntary hospital movement sweeping the country.[12] London saw the establishment of the Westminster (1719), Guy's (1721), St. George's (1733), The London (1740) and the Middlesex (1745). These were in addition to the ancient foundations of St. Bartholomew's (Bart's) in 1123 and St. Thomas's (Tommy's) in 1173, the year of canonisation of the martyred Thomas à Becket.[12]

8

At the instigation of the two most eminent and influential surgeons of the day, William Cheselden and John Ranby, a bill of separation received royal assent on 2 May 1745 despite the opposition of the barbers.[12] The surgeons departed and the barbers kept Barber-Surgeons Hall that was (and is) hyphenated and all the treasures except the Edward Arris Gift and the John Gale Annuity.[12] The Arris and Gale Lecture is still given annually at RCS England. The Hall in Monkwell Street was built by the Company of Barbers and completed in 1445. It was incinerated by the Great Fire of London that began on 2 September 1666 and replaced by 1674 (See Fig. 5)

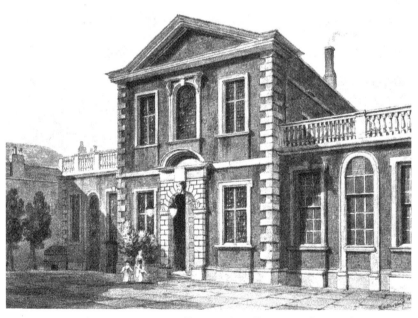

Figure 5. Barber-Surgeons' Hall, Monkwell Street dating from 1674 which replaced the original building completed in 1445 that was incinerated by the Great Fire in 1666. This Hall was almost completely rebuilt between 1864 and 1869 but was destroyed during the Blitz on 29 December 1940. Watercolour by George S. Shepherd, early nineteenth century.
Courtesy of the London Metropolitan Archives (City of London).

but almost completely rebuilt between 1864 and 1869.[13] This building was demolished by German bombs during the Blitz on 29 December 1940, rebuilt on a new site a short distance away in Monkwell Square and opened by the Queen Mother in 1969.[2]

John Ranby (1703-1773), elected a Fellow of the Royal Society (FRS) in 1724, had a large private practice and, in 1737, operated on Queen Caroline's strangulated umbilical hernia from which she succumbed at the age of 54! Ranby was a close friend and sergeant-surgeon to King George II (r. 1727-1760) and became the first master of the Company of Surgeons on 1 July 1745.[12] He was followed by William Cheselden, FRS (1688-1752) in 1746 who had been chosen as one of the two surgeon masters of the Company of Barbers and Surgeons in 1744.[12] He had qualified as a 'freeman' in 1711 and obtained an episcopal licence in 1712.[14] Cheselden, who specialised in 'surgery for stone' and ophthalmology, had been on the staff of St. Thomas's, the Westminster and St. George's. In 1738, he gave up his voluntary hospital posts to become surgeon to British Army pensioners at Chelsea Hospital now known as the Royal Hospital, Chelsea.[12] He was succeeded there by Ranby in 1752.[15] Interestingly, Cheselden's son-in-law, Charles Cotes, MP, DM (Oxon), FRCP (?-1748) was chairman of the parliamentary committee appointed to consider the merits of the case for separation.[12] After his first mastership, John Ranby presented a silver 'loving cup' to the company that is still in use by RCS England as a table decoration.[12] Ranby's apprentices paid a binding fee of £210 (£53,743)[9] but the Statute of Artificers, 1562 (5 Eliz.1 c.4) known as the 'Statute of Apprentices' had limited each master to three.[10]

The Court of Assistants of the Company of Surgeons held its first meeting on 1 July 1745 at Stationers' Hall in Ave Maria Lane when John Ranby was confirmed as the first master.[10] To this day, a newly elected president of RCS England takes office in July but now on a triennial basis. The Worshipful Company of Stationers provided accommodation (for a fee) until Surgeons' Hall (See Fig. 6) on the east side of the Old Bailey was completed in 1752 at

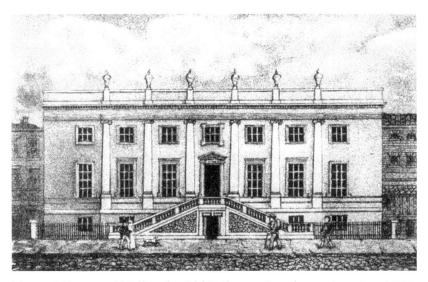

Figure 6. Surgeons' Hall at the Old Bailey, unsigned aquatint, circa 1752. The door beneath the stairs was used to transport bodies of publicly executed criminals into the Lecture Theatre for dissection. The building was completed in 1752.
William Jones, surveyor/architect.
Courtesy of the Archives of the Royal College of Surgeons of England.

a cost of £3,555 (£822,572)[9].[16] It was designed by the surveyor to the new company, William Jones.[16] A 100 years' lease of a plot of land adjacent to Newgate Prison had been acquired from the City of London.[12] The Hall was conveniently located to receive its annual quota of four bodies of publicly executed criminals for dissection in its large, well-appointed lecture theatre because there was a bizarre legal requirement that dissections take place within 400 yards of the prison. The Act of Separation laid down that a Court of Assistants of 21 (including a master and two wardens) was to be chosen by seniority for life.[17] An additional seven members were selected, also by seniority for life to form, with the *ex officio* master and two wardens, a 10 member Court of Examiners.[17]

Changes to the bye-laws in April 1748 codified the company's separation from the functions of a city livery company and

11

stipulated that the Court of Assistants should meet every month although they rarely did so.[17] Thus, the company was under the control of the master who continued to rotate annually, two wardens and seven examiners who, like the assistants, were required 'to continue in their office for and during their natural lives.'[17] Both courts were empowered to 'self-elect' any necessary replacements![17]

In 1629, King Charles I (r. 1625-1649) codified an order, originally issued in 1606, that had granted the surgeon members of the Company of Barbers and Surgeons the unremunerated privilege of examining Royal Navy, British Army and East India Company surgeons, approving their instrument chests and assessing the expenses of wounded officers and their claims for disability pensions.[6] After the separation in 1745, this duty became the responsibility of the Court of Examiners of the Company of Surgeons.[6]

In 1790, the demitting master, John Gunning, conceded in a philippic that the lucrative examinations (10s. 6d. per diploma for each examiner, approximately £115 in today's money)[9] were well-conducted. 'He then criticised the administration under six headings: the business of the two Courts, the Hall, the servants, the charities, the teaching and the library.'[17] For example, there were no books in the library that was used by the clerk as an office with the committee room as his 'eating parlour;' no lectures in the lecture theatre; no prepared specimens for teaching; mismanaged company finances and no charities.[17] Gunning did not acknowledge his own responsibility and declined to help 'improve matters.'[17]

Gunning's report was accepted and some administrative reforms were made but the Hall continued to be used almost exclusively for the organisation and conduct of examinations.[17] Students preferred to enroll in the established schools of anatomy and surgery in London most of which used the services of the 'resurrectionists' or 'body snatchers.'[18]

In 1796, the Court of Examiners put the Hall up for sale and two large houses, Nos. 41 and 42, on the south side of Lincoln's Inn Fields were identified of which the former was on the market.[19] Despite this usurpation of power, the Court of Assistants approved.[19] The Hall was in a state of disrepair and had never been frequented by practising surgeons who probably found the Old Bailey uncongenial with public executions drawing large crowds to Newgate Prison which continued until 1868. The prison was demolished in 1902 and replaced by the Central Criminal Court opened by King Edward VII (r. 1901-1910) in 1907. There was also a desire for complete separation from the archaic practices of City livery companies and moving west to Holborn enabled the company to acquire freehold property.[19] In 1796, Surgeons' Hall was 'sold to the Directors of the Court of Lieutenancy of the City Militia' for £2,000 (£240,640)[9] and used, initially, as a barracks.[19] In the same year, an offer of £5,500 (£661,760)[9] was accepted for vacant possession of No. 41 Lincoln's Inn Fields and the first Court of Assistants meeting was held there on 5 January 1797.[19]

On 1 March 1798, Rear-Admiral Sir Horatio Nelson (1758–1805) attended the Court of Examiners at No. 41 because of an infected amputation stump following fracture of his right humerus by a musket ball at Tenerife. He was awarded £135 1s. 0d. (£18,458)[9] for expenses.[6]

In 1799, H.M. Treasury paid £15,000 (£1.823 million)[9] for the extraordinary collection of 13,682 specimens and preparations illustrating comparative anatomy, pathology, osteology and natural history assembled by the Scottish anatomist, master surgeon and founder of scientific surgery, John Hunter, FRS (1728-1793).[20] The collection was placed in the care of the Company of Surgeons.[20]

From 1748, John Hunter's training included 11 years of assisting at the school of anatomy and surgery owned by his elder brother, William, in Covent Garden that moved to Jermyn Street in 1755 and Great Windmill Street in 1769. William Hunter, MD (Glasgow), LRCP (London), FRS, (1714-1788) was a physician, the leading obstetrician of his day and 'master of anatomy' at the Company of Surgeons from 1752. He was required by the RCP to sever his connection with the Company of Surgeons prior to acquiring the LRCP and, in 1756, incurred a 'fine of 40 guineas' (£9,718)[9] for doing so![17]

William arranged apprenticeships for John with William Cheselden at Chelsea Hospital from 1749 to 1750; with Percivall Pott (1714-1788) at Bart's from 1751 to 1754 followed by a post as the sole house surgeon, at St. George's. Interestingly, there is no mention of an indentured apprenticeship.[20] In 1761, during the Seven Years' War (1756-1763), John managed to obtain an appointment as an army surgeon and served on 'Belle Isle' off the coast of France where he obtained material for his magnificent *'Treatise on the Blood, Inflammation and Gun-Shot Wounds,'* eventually published in 1794. He was transferred to Portugal after a year on 'Belle Isle' where, needless to say, he studied the natural history and geology of the country. After the 'Peace of Paris' in 1763 he set up in private practice in Golden Square, Soho and, in 1764, acquired the Earl's Court House estate in Earl's Court Lane (now Road) located opposite the present-day eastern entrance to Earl's Court Underground Station. This was where he prepared, studied and kept most of his specimens along with an exotic menagerie! Earl's Court House was demolished in 1886.[20]

John Hunter was elected FRS in 1767 (Copley Medal 1787) and honorary surgeon to St. George's Hospital in 1768 shortly after acquiring the required diploma of the Company of Surgeons at the advanced age of 40![20] He was appointed sergeant-surgeon to King George III (r. 1760-1820) in 1776; elected to the *'Académie Royale de Chirurgie de Paris'* in 1783; the 'American Philosophical Society' in 1787 and appointed surgeon-general to the British Army in 1790 by the Prime Minister, William Pitt the Younger (See Fig. 7).[20] Sadly John Hunter, who was known to suffer from angina, died prematurely at the age of 65 from an acute coronary

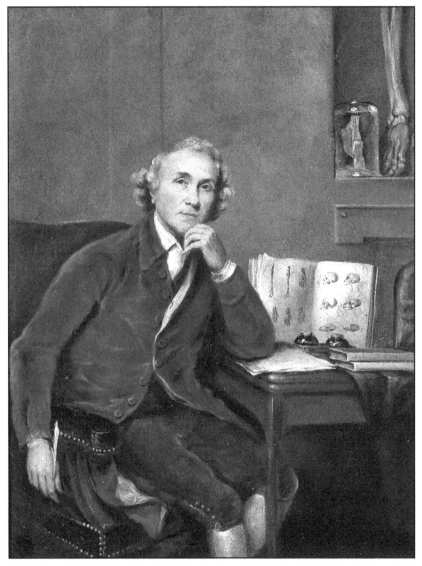

Figure 7. John Hunter, FRS (1728-1793), London-based Scottish anatomist, master surgeon and founder of scientific surgery. Oil painting after Sir Joshua Reynolds, PRA (1723-1792). John Hunter, in 1786, reflecting on the future of surgery!
Courtesy of the Wellcome Collection.

occlusion. It is alleged to have been caused by a row with the Board of Governors of St. George's Hospital over two of his students who had not been approved to work in the hospital as Hunter's apprentices.[20] From 1859, his remains have rested in the north aisle of the nave of Westminster Abbey having been moved from the vaults of St. Martin-in-the-Fields where he was interred in 1793.

After the sale of the collection, most of Hunter's catalogues, manuscripts, correspondence and notes were removed in a cart by acting executor, surgeon Sir Everard Home, PPRCS, FRS (1756-1832) with the approval of his sister Anne, John Hunter's widow. The pretext used was that this was Hunter's wish because the material was 'not fit for publication.'[20] John and Anne Hunter (née Home, 1742-1821) married in 1771 and had two surviving children (of four), John Banks and Agnes Margaretta. Anne Hunter was a well-known intellectual and lyrical poet some of whose work was set to music by Joseph Haydn (1732-1809) who had been treated by her husband in 1791. These included six of the 12 'English Canzonettas' and 'O Tuneful Voice' composed in 1802. Haydn's frequent meetings with the attractive widow in London in 1794-95 led to speculation about their relationship! The musicologist H. C. Robbins Landon (1926-2009) confirmed that Anne's libretto for 'The Creation' postdated its composition in 1797-98. It was discovered in the archives of RCS England in 1990 included in the 'Baillie Hunter Papers.' Everard Home had worked closely with John Hunter, initially as his assistant, and it is now established that he published much of Hunter's research as his own work over a period of 23 years including an astonishing 92 papers in Philosophical Transactions of the Royal Society.[20]

In 1823, Home incinerated the documents, presumably to avoid exposure, causing a chimney fire at his home whilst continuing to insist that this was John Hunter's wish! Fortunately, most of the destroyed material had been copied by William Clift, FRS (1775-1849), who had been hired by Hunter's widow in 1793 to care for the collections at Earls Court House and the spacious premises at 28 Leicester Square (purchased leasehold in 1783) until their sale in 1799 and removal to Lincoln's Inn Fields in 1806.[20] It was comparison of Home's publications with Clift's copies of Hunter's originals that confirmed Home as an unprincipled plagiarist! Subsequently, Clift, became the first 'Conservator' of the Hunterian Museum.[20] The old buildings at No. 28 on the east side of Leicester Square were demolished in 1897.[20] John Hunter's bust was removed during the redesign of the square in 2012 and its whereabouts are unknown.

V   The Royal Charter of 1800
The Royal College of Surgeons in London

On 22 March 1800, the Great Seal was affixed to the royal charter granted by King George III creating the Royal College of Surgeons in London and the Court of Assistants held its first meeting on 10 April 1800.[21] In 1802, No. 42 became available and was acquired as a stopgap 'Hunterian Museum' for £4,100 (£425,268)[9].[21] Ironically, No. 42 had once been the home of former Lord Chancellor, Lord Thurlow (1731-1806), who had asserted during a diatribe against the company in the House of Lords on 10 April 1797 that, 'there is no more science in surgery than in butchery.'[22] Lord Thurlow's intervention killed the first attempt to establish a college of surgeons by Act of Parliament. Shaw (2012) suggests that the unmarried Thurlow's 'rejection in marriage by a surgeon's daughter' in his youth might explain his animus.[22] Belatedly, the company's lawyers discovered that 'irregular' proceedings, by the Courts of Assistants and Examiners in 1796, had resulted in 'the *ipso facto* dissolution of the company.'[19] Thus, there was no longer a legal requirement to risk the failure of a second bill in Parliament and the company was able to secure a royal charter by means of a 'Petition to the Sovereign in Council.'[19]

In 1806, after years of dithering over funding, a grant from the Treasury of £15,000 (£1.432 million)[9] resulted in a decision to demolish Nos. 41 and 42 and construct an imposing building designed by George Dance the Younger (1741-1825), which was to include a purpose-built museum for the Hunterian collection.[21] The building was not completed until 1813 following an additional grant from the Treasury of £12,500 (£1.044 million)[9] in 1810 that had been requested by the college.[21] Much of the additional funding was required for the construction of a Portland stone neo-classical portico which the surgeons were unwilling to forgo despite the architect's advice.[21] Clearly, they regarded it as a symbol of their newly-acquired professional status (See Fig. 8)! Between 1800 and 1813 there were only two courses of lectures, on comparative anatomy by Sir Everard Home in 1810 and on surgery by Sir William Blizard (1743-1835) in the same year.[21]

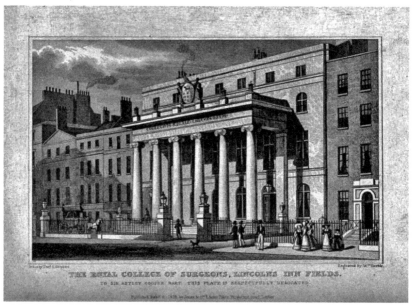

Figure 8. The Royal College of Surgeons in London, 41-42 Lincoln's Inn Fields, engraving by Wm. Deeble after Thomas H. Shepherd 1828. Construction began in 1806 but was not completed until 1813. George Dance the Younger, architect. Courtesy of the Wellcome Collection.

VI   The Royal College of Surgeons in London
The Royal Charter of 1822

Changes had been proposed to the constitution of the new college and on 22 February 1822 King George IV (r. 1820-1830) issued a supplemental charter allowing control by a President, two Vice Presidents and a Council that replaced the Court of Assistants but with no changes to the electoral system.[23] The last master and first president from 1 July 1821 was Sir Everard Home followed by Sir William Blizard on 1 July 1822, Council was to choose office-holders, each year, from amongst their number and the Court of Examiners would continue as before.[23] The King took the opportunity to present and authorise the use of a mace engraved with the 'Arms of the College surmounted by the Royal Arms' that still features on ceremonial occasions.[23] Council decided, after criticism of the drab appearance of Sir Everard Home at the coronation on 19 July 1821, that a 'more splendid gown' should be worn by the President on 'very special occasions.'[23]

Following separation from the barbers in 1745, the Company of Surgeons found itself without a coat of arms.[24] Rather than incur the expense of presenting a 'memorial' to the Earl Marshal of England, the company paid a man named Brookshead three guineas (£757)[9] to design a new one.[25] The original and the current coat of arms feature the two sons of Asclepius (Greek god of medicine and son of Apollo) who were surgeons at the siege of Troy. In 293 BC the cult spread to Rome where Asclepius was worshipped as Aesculapius.[25]

In recognition of the King's gift of a mace, the college added a crown and mace to the eagle regardant (a symbol of fortitude) to indicate royal status that became the official logo of the college.[25] In compliance with a Royal Warrant dated 17 September 1822, the 'College of Arms' issued letters patent granting armorial bearings to the college. Brookshead's original design was modified with the addition of a 'Lion of England' and the Cross of St.

George bearing a crown but was otherwise unchanged.[25] The motto, 'QUAE PROSUNT OMNIBUS ARTES' translates as 'The Arts which are of Service to All' (See Fig. 9).[25]

Within twenty years, Dance's building had become structurally unsound and was considered too small for the Hunterian Collection.[24] House No. 40 had been purchased in 1830 and a new

Coat of Arms of the Royal College of Surgeons of England

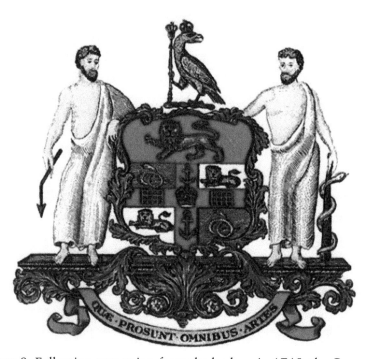

Figure 9. Following separation from the barbers in 1745, the Company of Surgeons was without a coat of arms and a replacement was designed by a Mr. Brookshead at a cost of three guineas. In compliance with a Royal Warrant issued by King George IV in September 1822, the 'College of Arms' issued letters patent granting armorial bearings to the college. Brookshead's design was modified by the addition of a 'Lion of England' and the 'Cross of St. George bearing a Crown.' (See pages 19 and 20) Courtesy of the Archives of the Royal College of Surgeons of England.

building had been designed by the winner of a competition in 1833, Sir Charles Barry (1795-1860), who became a Fellow of the Royal Institute of British Architects (FRIBA) on its foundation in 1834.[26] He had just completed 'The Travellers Club' and went on to win the competition in 1836, with the assistance of Augustus Pugin (1812-1852), to rebuild the 'Palace of Westminster' (Houses of Parliament) after its destruction by fire in 1834. Pugin subsequently designed furnishings, statuary, stained glass, decorative floor tiles and mosaics until his mental breakdown and death in 1852.

VII The Royal College of Surgeons in London
The 'Barry' building 1836

George Dance's building was demolished in 1834 but Sir Charles Barry had been contracted, against his wishes, to preserve the portico.[27] He was permitted to modify the entablature by removing the inscription '*Collegium Regale Chirurgorum*;' the coat of arms and the four lanterns. Its position for symmetry was adjusted by moving a column from west to east and the six Ionic columns were fluted.[27] Barry surmounted the new structure with a Portland stone carved cornice and frieze that was inscribed, '*Aedes Collegii Chirurgorum Londinensis - Diplomate Regio Corporati. A.D. MDCCC*' that translates as '*Temple of the London College of Surgeons - Royal Corporation for Diplomates. AD. 1800.*'[25] The building was completed in 1836 at a cost of £45,000 (£5.469 million)[9] exceeding the original estimate by £27,000 (£3.281 million)[9].[26] Sir Charles gave a detailed explanation to Council and an acrimonious meeting concluded with warmest congratulations to Barry on his 'splendid work' (See Fig. 10)![2]

VIII The Royal Charter of 1843
The Royal College of Surgeons of England

On 14 September 1843, the Royal College of Surgeons of England was created by royal charter granted by Queen Victoria

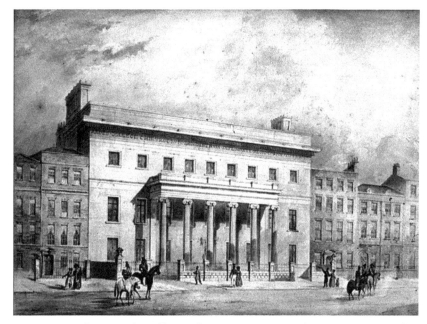

Figure 10. The Royal College of Surgeons in London, 40-42 Lincoln's Inn Fields, watercolour by Frederick Rumble 1836. The original building by George Dance was demolished in 1834 with the exception of the portico and the 'Barry' building was completed in 1836.
Sir Charles Barry, FRIBA, architect.
Courtesy of the Archives of the Royal College of Surgeons of England.

(r. 1837-1901).[28] *'Londinensis'* was replaced by *'Anglici' (English)* and the inscription remains unchanged to this day.[28] Mindful of the possibility of future expansion, the college continued to acquire adjacent properties as they came on the market - No. 39 in 1834, 37 in 1847, 43 in 1860, 44 in 1867 and 38 in 1875.[26] Between 1851 and 1855, Barry supervised various interior modifications and extensions southward towards Portugal Street, often related to the Hunterian Museum.[26]

When Sir Charles Barry died in 1860, Stephen Salter, FRIBA (1825-1896) became architect to the college. Between 1888 and 1891, he extended the Barry building on to the sites of No. 39 to the east and No. 43 to the west whilst preserving the façade at a cost of £19,000 (£2.569 million)[9].[29] The imposing library was lengthened eastward beyond the fireplace and two stories were added above Barry's cornice.[27] The new wings and floors were surmounted by Portland stone balustrades. No. 39 in the east was nine feet narrower than No. 43 in the west and the difference was utilised in the interior of the latter.[27] The extra nine feet of the façade of No. 43 was, and still is, identifiable externally and initially was modified to harmonise with No. 44 (See Figs. 1 & 11).[27] 'The portion of the façade within the portico and most of the architectural features are composed of artificial stones, i.e. cast blocks of concrete and stucco.'[27] 'The remainder of the front is faced with stucco.'[27] It is this façade and library which survives to the present day. The cost was defrayed with a small portion of the magnificent legacy of Sir Erasmus Wilson, PPRCS, FRS (1809-1884), of £200,000 (£27.660 million)[9].[26] The only other significant remodelling before the Second World War was the

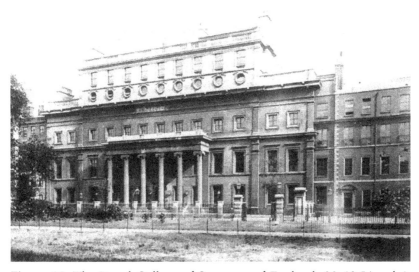

Figure 11. The Royal College of Surgeons of England, 39-43 Lincoln's Inn Fields and house nos. 38 and 44, photograph 1899. The extensions were completed in 1891.
Stephen Salter, FRIBA, architect.
Courtesy of the Archives of the Royal College of Surgeons of England.

conversion, in 1936, of the upper floors of the building into three floors of laboratory space.[26]

IX   Diploma of the Royal College of Surgeons in London 1800 to 1843

For centuries, surgeons had conducted the mandatory *viva voce* licensing examination after the required seven-year indentured apprenticeship *(vide supra)*. In 1800, following the foundation of the Royal College of Surgeons in London, the examination to acquire a licence to practise cost 20 guineas (£1,871)[9] and the diploma became known as Membership of the Royal College of Surgeons in London (MRCS).[6] A written paper was only required of doubtful MRCS candidates until 1860, when written and clinical components were introduced.[6]

Candidates complained that there was no written curriculum until one finally appeared in 1819 requiring certification of education and training.[6] In 1824, the Examiners issued a regulation that 'the only Schools of Surgery recognized by the Court be those of London, Dublin, Edinburgh, Glasgow and Aberdeen.'[6] This caused a furore because the newly-founded provincial medical schools in Birmingham, Bristol, Leeds, Liverpool, Manchester, Newcastle/Durham and Sheffield were excluded.[6] The apothecaries had already inspected and approved these schools for training in general medicine *(vide infra)*.[6] Five years were to pass before this contentious regulation was abrogated and it is evident that, by this time, the old-style indentured apprenticeship was falling into disuse.[6]

Unfortunately, a dispute with the physician of the navy, the surgeon-general of the army and the surgeon-general of the East India Company, that had caused problems for several decades, came to a head because the new college continued to assert that military surgeons were examined to a lower standard, at a cost of five guineas (£446),[9] than their civilian counterparts.[6] They were not licensed to practise surgery when they returned to civilian life unless they passed the civilian MRCS at a cost of 20 guineas (£1,871)[9].[6] The military authorities responded by accepting licensing qualifications from the 'Schools of Surgery in Aberdeen, Dublin, Edinburgh, and Glasgow' in addition to London but, by 1843, applicant military surgeons were being examined only by the medical departments of their respective services.[6]

Subsequently, the apothecaries (vide infra) decided to examine retired military doctors who wished to enter civilian practice as physicians free of charge and awarded the Licentiate of the Society of Apothecaries (LSA) qualification to successful candidates.[6] Those who wanted to practise surgery were still required to pay 20 guineas to take the civilian MRCS but the college did agree to grant the diploma, without examination (or charge), to surgeons who had served in the Napoleonic Wars (1803 to 1815).[6]

X Diplomas of the Royal College of Surgeons of England from 1843

The royal charter of 14 September 1843 created the diploma of Fellow of the Royal College of Surgeons of England (FRCS) exclusively for specialist surgeons that was to be quite distinct from the qualifying MRCS.[28] It was to be acquired by examination after a one year period during which members of the college, with specific exclusions, were to be elected FRCS ad eundem based on their 'surgical, scientific and general distinction.'[30] 300 were to be chosen within the first three months and additional names added thereafter.[28] It was, of course, impossible to please everyone and Council was deluged with complaints from members who had been overlooked and from Sir William Burnett, Physician of the Navy and Sir James McGrigor, Surgeon-General of the Army who each submitted lists containing a total of about 400 names.[28] Council protested and the lists were modified![28] In addition to military and East India Company surgeons, the great majority of the 10,000 general practitioners held both the LSA and the MRCS as 'physicians and surgeons.' The MRCS was the usual surgical qualification in England and Wales but not required by statute law until the Medical Act of 1858.[30] Thus the total number of aggrieved members may have been as high as 20,000 and less than 600 had been elected to the fellowship![30]

Candidates for the new FRCS examination had to be 'twenty-five years of age, of certified good character and to have passed six years in professional study.'[28] At least, three years in a recognised London hospital and one year as a house surgeon or dresser in an approved English hospital were required. For those with an arts degree the period of study was reduced to five years. 'Each candidate had to write and send in an account of six clinical cases he had observed.'[28] The first FRCS examination took place in December 1844 and a fee of 10 guineas (£1,419)[9] was payable for an examination in two parts separated by one day. The first part (primary) on 3 December was in anatomy and physiology and the second part (final) on 5 December was in surgery, pathology and therapeutics consisting of a 'written paper (on which the candidate was questioned), dissections and operations.' 24 candidates were successful and it was decided to hold the next examination in April 1845.[28]

The final FRCS was not an exit diploma. It comprised 'surgery-in-general' and had a pass rate of circa 25 per cent which was unchanged until the old-style FRCS was replaced in 2004. It was required at registrar/resident surgeon level as evidence of suitability for higher surgical training (HST).[2] Eligibility criteria were modified as necessary and complied with a succession of Medical Acts of Parliament. In the 1970s, the primary FRCS could be taken after the preregistration year (internship) introduced in 1953. Requirements for the final examination were six months in accident and emergency, six months in a preferred specialty and 18 months in general surgery.[2]

In the mid-twentieth century, there were bottlenecks at registrar to senior registrar and senior registrar to consultant levels that might have been eased by thoughtful planning and increasing the number of senior posts as an expensive alternative to the exploitation of surgeons-in-training. It could take years to become a senior registrar and many more to secure a consultant appointment in a chosen field. Registrars with the FRCS and years of clinical, operative and research experience, publications and higher degrees who were unable to progress within a reasonable time frame, tended to emigrate to Australia, Canada. New Zealand or the United States. They were replaced by international medical graduates many of whom were obliged to accept permanent sub-consultant, staff grade posts. This was unconscionable in view of the development of specialties such as cardiothoracic, trauma and orthopaedics, maxillofacial, neurosurgery, paediatric surgery, plastic surgery and urology as well-defined, specialist areas of practice.

Women were not admitted to the college until 1909 and not allowed to vote or stand for election to Council.[6] The first MRCS was Dossibai Patell (1881-1960) from Bombay (now Mumbai) in 1910 and the first FRCS was Eleanor Davies-Colley (1874-1934), in 1911, who had trained at The London (Royal Free Hospital) School of Medicine for Women in the Gray's Inn Road that moved to Pond Street, Hampstead in 1974. The hospital was founded in 1828 by William Marsden, (1796-1867) who qualified MRCS in 1826 and went on to establish what became the Royal Marsden Hospital (for cancer) in 1851. Restrictions on women were not removed until 1926.[6]

XI Eligibility for a Council Seat from 1843

Council was increased in number to 24 by the charter of 1843 to be elected, in person, by and from the fellows who were eligible for a Council seat provided that they had not been involved in the practice of pharmacy or midwifery during the previous five years. The latter requirement was abrogated by a supplemental charter in 1852.[31] The term of office was limited to eight years and the three most senior members would retire each year but eligibility for re-election was to be unlimited.[31] The 10 member Court of Examiners was to be elected by and from Council or from the fellows and was to retain office 'during the pleasure of Council.'[31] Thus, the controversial practice of tenure for life had been almost, but not quite, abolished!

XII   Thomas Wakley, MP, MRCS (1795-1862)

Much of the credit for the changes to the constitution of the college must be given to Thomas Wakley, who qualified MRCS (in London) in 1817 although he believed that they did not go far enough and was to be disappointed in his lifetime. He is described as being 'well-equipped with dauntless courage, political sagacity and reforming zeal' and was a highly effective speaker and writer.[6] He was founding editor of *The Lancet* in 1823 and become a Member of Parliament in 1835. Wakley enjoyed denouncing the college's undemocratic, governing gerontocracy and vigorously supported younger surgeons who wished to have more say in the conduct of affairs.[6]

Wakley would be pleased to know that enfranchisement of members was eventually achieved in the early twenty-first century following the transformation of the MRCS into the Intercollegiate MRCS that now marks the end of the first stage of specialist training *(vide infra)*. The impediment was that members of the college were not regarded as specialist surgeons. Their inferior status was affirmed by a bye-law requiring that they use the back door in Portugal Street to enter the building rather than the impressive front entrance in Lincoln's Inn Fields that was reserved for Council, the Court of Examiners and the fellows![6] Since 1815, their plight had been exacerbated by the Apothecaries Act and, ultimately, by the Medical Act of 1886 *(vide infra)*.

XIII   The Court of Assistants, Council and Innovation from 1800

Younger surgeons were concerned about the obstetrical disasters presided over by unlettered and untrained midwives.[6] Continuous pressure had been applied to Council by the London Obstetrical Society to introduce training and a licensing qualification.[6] This organisation was comprised of both physicians and surgeons with an interest who were often discriminated against by medical colleagues who considered the practice of obstetrics to be demeaning. [6]

In 1827, President of the Royal College of Physicians for 24 years, baronet Sir Henry Halford, DM (Oxon), PRCP, FRS, GCH (1766–1844), wrote to Sir Robert Peel (1788-1850), Home Secretary at the time, stating that in his view, 'midwifery is an act foreign to the habits of a gentleman of enlarged academic education.'[6] As late as 1834, Sir Anthony Carlisle, FRCS, FRS (1768-1840), Member of Council, declared that it was an 'imposture to pretend that a medical man is required at a labour.'[6]

It is astonishing that the highly educated husbands, fathers and grandfathers who controlled the medical royal colleges in London could have believed that childbirth was a purely natural process at which skilled intervention was never required.[6] The pressure became intense and a Diploma in Midwifery was instituted in December 1842 for medically qualified men.[6] Midwives were trained and examined informally by the London Obstetrical Society until the Midwives Act became law in 1902.[6]

It was anticipated that the conservative Council would oppose the introduction of obstetrical anaesthesia in 1847 by Scottish obstetrician James Young Simpson (1811-1870), created baronet in 1866, on both medical and moral grounds.[6] However, it is well-known that Queen Victoria delivered her eighth child, Prince Leopold, in 1853 after inhaling chloroform via a silk handkerchief for nearly an hour under the supervision of Dr. John Snow (1813-1858), 'the world's first anaesthetist.'[6] The Queen is believed to have described the experience as 'delightful beyond measure...' and repeated it in 1857 with Princess Beatrice. Dr. Snow was heavily criticised, particularly by *The Lancet*, but was not identified and Council, for once, refrained from comment.[6]

In 1854, Dr. Snow had further impressed The Queen and Prince Albert by correctly linking the cholera outbreak, in Soho, to contaminated water from the Broad Street (now Broadwick Street) pump.[6] After he had the handle removed, new cases immediately diminished. Sadly, he died of a stroke at the early age of 45.[6] John Snow, a teetotaler, is the only English physician to have a public house (pub) named after him that is located in Broadwick Street! A replica pump without a handle stands outside the pub in its original position!

In the spring of 1867, Joseph Lister, FRCS, PRS (1827-1912), Regius Professor of Surgery at the University of Glasgow, published a series of papers in *The Lancet* on antisepsis using carbolic acid (phenol); the most significant and revolutionary advance in medical science of the nineteenth century.[6] They were based on the seminal work on fermentation, putrefaction and microorganisms by Professor Louis Pasteur (1822-1895) the 'father of microbiology,' working in Lille and then in Paris, that were published between 1860 and 1864. Lister himself, knighted and later the first surgeon to be elevated to the peerage, regarded asepsis as a logical modification of his antisepsis but was doubtful of its efficacy.[6] Antisepsis was embraced by the younger generation of surgeons throughout Europe, the UK and the US with astonishing reductions in morbidity and mortality.[6] Unsurprisingly, it is recorded that Council 'either did not credit the reports or belittled them.'[6]

Lister, who had held the chairs of surgery in both Edinburgh and Glasgow, accepted the chair at King's College London in 1877. He felt that a London base would be helpful in his campaign to persuade his elderly critics of the efficacy of his techniques most of whom were unconvinced by the 'germ-theory' of disease and preferred the 'miasma theory' originally propounded by Hippocrates and Galen and still in vogue at the time. Lister became irritated by the obtuseness of Council of which he was a member and did not stand for re-election eventually becoming President of the much more prestigious Royal Society. This body, founded in 1660 as 'The Royal Society of London for Improving Natural Knowledge,' consists entirely of fellows elected by peer review who have made substantial contributions in all areas of science, mathematics, engineering and medicine. Today, there are 1,400 fellows of whom 69 are Nobel Laureates. The 'miasma theory' persisted until 1876 when German physician Robert Koch (1843-1910), the 'father of medical bacteriology,' proved conclusively that anthrax was caused by the bacterium '*Bacillus anthracis.*'

Council's criticism of Lister's achievements is entirely analogous to the reaction expected from senior surgeons, who did not disappoint, regarding the revolutionary technique of laparoscopic cholecystectomy created by German surgeon, Dr. Erich Mühe, 120 years later that was the subject of derisive comments *(vide infra)*. For centuries, revolutionary advances in science and technology have been greeted with approval by some and angry dissent by others, often the most senior, whose body of work becomes subject to 'reassessment.'[6]

XIV   The Worshipful Society of Apothecaries

In 1704, the Worshipful Society of Apothecaries, (formed by royal charter in 1617 but in existence before 1316), won a key legal suit against the RCP in the appellate jurisdiction of the House of Lords, which ruled that apothecaries could both prescribe and dispense medicines after their five-year apprenticeship.[6] This decision led to the direct evolution of the apothecary into today's general practitioner.[6] An Act of Parliament in 1815 gave the apothecaries, the right to regulate the practice of general medicine throughout England and Wales, and to conduct the LSA qualifying examination.[6]

John Keats (1795-1821), after his apprenticeship from 1810 to 1815 and less than a year as a dresser at Guy's Hospital, presented himself for examination before the Court of Examiners on 26 July

31

1816 and became an LSA. He was already suffering from tuberculosis and, subsequently, devoted himself to becoming one of the most significant 'second generation' poets of the 'Romantic' era along with Lord Byron and Percy Bysshe Shelley who were his exact contemporaries. Sadly, he succumbed to the disease in Rome in 1821 at the age of only 25 but his legacy was sublime!

Surgery and midwifery were excluded from the LSA until the Medical Act of 1886 received royal assent. The qualification was renamed the Licentiate in Medicine and Surgery of the Society of Apothecaries (LMSSA) also by statute in 1907.[6] The examination was taken at the historic Apothecaries Hall in Black Friars Lane that had been rebuilt after the Great Fire in 1666.[2] The original building, parts of which survived, was the thirteenth century guesthouse of the Dominican Friary acquired by the Society in 1632.[2]

The tale of a candidate taking the LMSSA in the 1960s, probably apocryphal, circulated around the London medical school rugby clubs for years. He called the invigilator and asked for a pot of ale as prescribed in the regulations of 1815. A pint of bitter was duly supplied from a local pub. Some weeks later the Society exacted its revenge - he was fined £50 for not wearing his sword before the Court of Examiners!

General practitioners liked to describe themselves as 'physician and surgeon' and so, until 1886, they were obliged to hold both the LSA and the MRCS as evidenced by two annual publications: *The Medical Directory* dating from 1845 and *The Medical Register* from 1859.[6] Both are still in existence and available online.

The latter was published by the General Council of Medical Education and Registration of the United Kingdom now known as the General Medical Council (GMC) which was created by the landmark Medical Act of 1858.[6] Prior to 1858, the state of the law was intricate and obscure and almost anybody could set themselves up as a medical practitioner.[2] There were untrained, self-styled physicians, surgeons, bone setters, dentists and midwives in every town and village at a time when the scientific age of medicine was just beginning.[2] The GMC was made responsible for medical registration throughout the British Isles consisting, at the time, of Great Britain (England, Wales and Scotland), Ireland, the Hebrides, the Isles of Scilly, the Isle of Man, the Orkney Islands and the Shetland Islands.[6] It was empowered only to recommend disqualification to the Privy Council of any of the 19 licensing bodies active in 1858 that were considered to be substandard.[6] Nevertheless, the significant risk of harm or death due to widespread quackery was greatly reduced.

In the early 1880s, it became obvious to RCS England that many years of negotiations with the RCP, the apothecaries and the universities, in the hope of establishing a single portal of entry into the medical profession, had failed.[6] For this reason, the college agreed to cooperate with the RCP in offering, with the approval of the GMC, what became known as the Conjoint Diploma of LRCP, MRCS as a non-university qualification to practise medicine, surgery and midwifery in England and Wales.[2] RCS England had already instituted the aforementioned Diploma in Midwifery for medically-qualified men in December 1842.[6] The written, clinical and *viva voce* Conjoint examination, was to comprise chemistry, chemical physics, materia medica, medical botany, pharmacy, anatomy, physiology, pathology, medicine, surgery, midwifery, and forensic medicine.[2] The colleges planned to hold the first examination in January 1885 prior to completion of the new Examination Hall on the Embankment in 1887.[6] The Conjoint Diploma was confirmed by the Medical Act of 1886 to be a lawful qualification to practise medicine, surgery and midwifery throughout the British Isles.

XV   Examination Hall, 2 Savoy Place, 1887 to 1909

Examination Hall at Savoy Place on the Embankment just to the west of Waterloo Bridge was commissioned, jointly, by the RCP and RCS England. In 1884, a plot of land was leased for 99 years from the Duchy of Lancaster.[6] The building was designed by Stephen Salter (*vide supra*) to accommodate 600 candidates taking the non-university qualifying examination. The foundation stone was laid by, 'Victoria; Queen of Great Britain and Ireland; Empress of India... on 24 March 1886 in the presence of a distinguished and numerous company including a thousand doctors.'[6] The building was completed in 1887 at a cost of less than £25,000 (£3.497 million)[9] (See Fig. 12).[6] Between 1887 and 1889, the Hall was extended to include a lecture theatre, classrooms and laboratories in which luminaries, such as future Nobel Laureate (1932) C. S. Sherrington, OM, FRCS, FRCP, PRS (1857–1952), undertook research.[6] In 1892, work on the *typhoid bacillus* resulted in two deaths including the principal researcher, Dr Henry Tylden

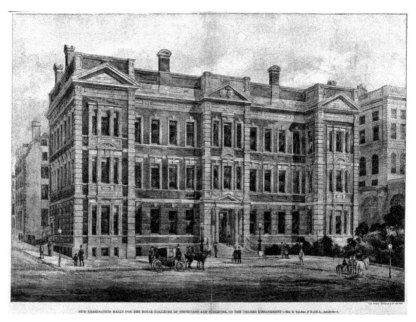

Figure 12. Examination Hall, 2 Savoy Place, lithograph 1888. The building was completed in 1887 and sold to the Institution of Electrical Engineers in 1909. The nascent BBC rented accommodation here from 1923 to 1932 on what became known to listeners as 'Savoy Hill.' Stephen Salter, FRIBA, architect.
Courtesy of the Wellcome Collection.

(1857-1892).[6] From 1894 to 1902, *anti-diphtheritic serum* was manufactured for the Metropolitan Asylums Board.[6]

In 1902, the colleges were offered an anonymous donation of £100,000 (£13.078 million)[9] to initiate cancer research.[6] The Cancer Research Fund was formed to develop a research programme and provided with laboratory space in Examination Hall. It became the Imperial Cancer Research Fund (ICRF) two years later and the relationship with RCS England continued for almost a century *(vide infra).*[6]

In 1909, the colleges decided to accept an offer of £50,000 (£6.332 million)[9] for the remaining lease of 74 years from the Institution of Electrical Engineers (IEE). Accommodation was rented to the nascent British Broadcasting Corporation (BBC) by the IEE between 1923 and 1932 on what became known to listeners as 'Savoy Hill'. The Institution of Engineering and Technology, formed by the merger of the IEE with the Institution of Incorporated Engineers in 2006, still leases the property from the Duke of Lancaster, His Majesty The King.

XVI Examination Hall, 8-11 Queen Square, 1912 to 1982

A neo-Wren style Examination Hall in Queen Square, designed by Andrew Prentice, FRIBA (1866-1941), was built at a cost of £31,644 (£3.845 million)[9] and ready for occupation in May 1912 (See Fig. 13).[6] Until that time, the colleges and the ICRF remained at Savoy Place by courtesy of the IEE. In 1963, ICRF transferred to a purpose-built research facility at Nos. 44-46 Lincoln's Inn Fields abutting the college to the west (See Fig. 3). The vacated laboratory space in Queen Square was used by RCS England's Department of Pharmacology until 1982 when the building was sold to the National Hospital for Neurology and Neurosurgery for £1,375 million (£5.163 million)[9] after the colleges acquired the freehold.[32] The various examinations were moved to the premises of the two colleges.

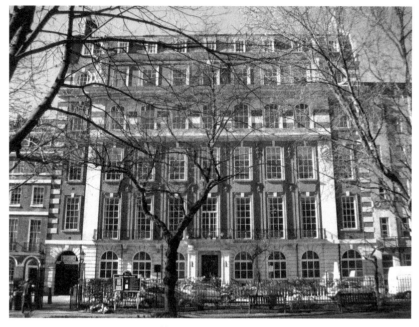

Figure 13. Examination Hall, 8-11 Queen Square completed in 1912 and sold to the National Hospital for Neurology and Neurosurgery in 1982. Andrew N. Prentice, FRIBA, architect
Photographed by the author, 16 October 2016.

ICRF became 'Cancer Research UK' in 2002 and amalgamated with the Medical Research Council's (MRC) 'Francis Crick Institute' in St. Pancras in 2015. The LSE bought the site in 2013 and demolished the ICRF building in 2018. The £145 million, 10 story Marshall Building (plus two basement levels), the LSE's largest establishment, now abuts the college to the west (See Fig. 14) and completes the eclectic range of architectural styles on the south side of Lincoln's Inn Fields!

In summary, the original MRCS was offered for 85 years from 1800 to 1885, the Conjoint Diploma for 116 years from 1885 until its abolition by the GMC in 2001 along with the LSA/ LMSSA in 2003 that had survived for 188 years. From the beginning of the twenty-first century, entry into the medical

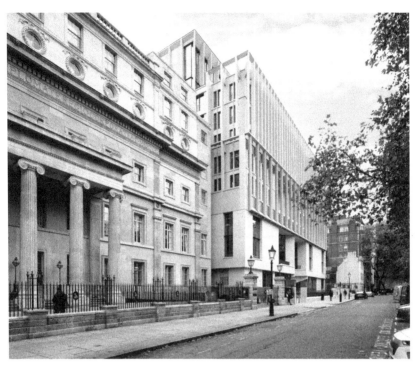

Figure 14. The London School of Economics' Marshall Building, 44-46 Lincoln's Inn Fields abutting RCS England, photograph 11 November 2021. Grafton Architects, Dublin.
Courtesy of fotohaus ltd.

profession in the UK was open only to graduates holding a medical degree awarded by a recognised university.'[6]

The Conjoint Diploma and the LMSSA remained popular until their abolition. Overseas graduates used them as a qualification to practise in the UK without further ado until the introduction of the Professional and Linguistic Assessments Board (PLAB) in 1978.[6] British students based in London regarded them as a practice run and an insurance policy against failing their qualifying university degrees.[6] British candidates who had trained at prestigious universities in Europe because they were unable to secure a place at medical school in the UK took one of the examinations in order to practise in their home country.[6]

XVII   The Second World War and its Aftermath

In the early hours of 11 May 1941, the Blitz caused severe damage to the college building (See Fig. 15).[33] Adjoining houses Nos. 35 to 38 on the eastern side were more or less demolished behind their façades by incendiaries and high explosive bombs (See Fig. 16).[33] House No. 38 had been used to display part of the Hunterian Museum Collection but, despite safe storage of valued items elsewhere and adequate air raid precautions, about two-fifths of John Hunter's original collection was destroyed (See Fig. 17).[33] The college operated from Examination Hall in Queen Square until temporary arrangements could be made in less damaged parts of the college.[33]

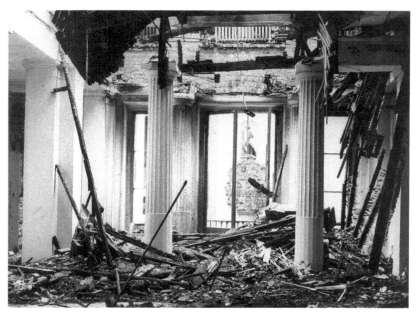

Figure 15. The inner hall of the Royal College of Surgeons of England (See Fig. 17) damaged by the Blitz on 11 May 1941, photograph late May 1941. The rebuilt college was opened, formally, by Her Majesty Queen Elizabeth II, accompanied by The Duke of Edinburgh, on 7 November 1962.
Courtesy of the Archives of the Royal College of Surgeons of England.

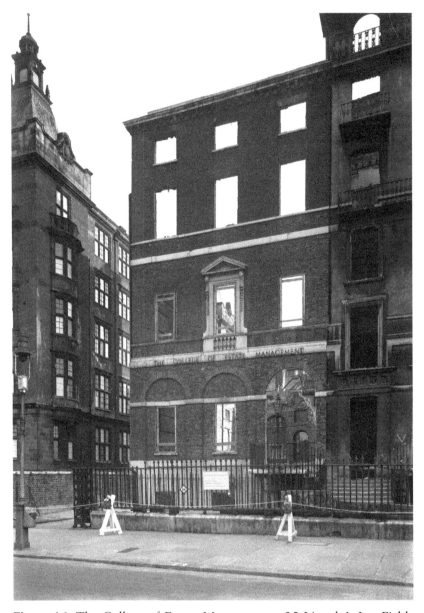

Figure 16. The College of Estate Management, 35 Lincoln's Inn Fields after the Blitz on 11 May 1941, photograph late 1941.
Sir Robert Taylor, architect, 1754.
Courtesy of Architectural Press Archive / RIBA Collections

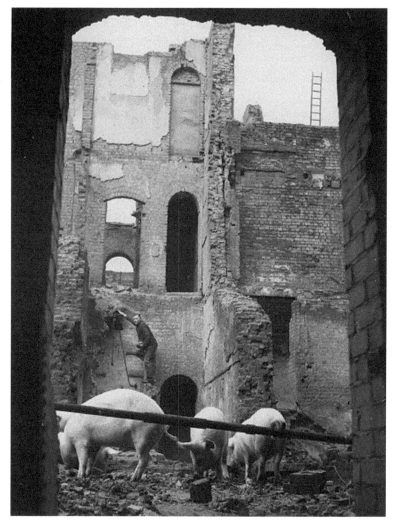

Figure 17. No. 38 Lincoln's Inn Fields which contained part of the Hunterian Museum Collection destroyed by the Blitz on 11 May 1941. The National Fire Service was permitted to raise pigs, rabbits and chickens until the end of the war, This photograph was published in *Picture Post* on 3 April 1943.
Courtesy of Hulton Deutsch / Getty Images.

Council saw an opportunity to extend RCS England's ownership of land to the east of the college by acquiring the bomb-sites of Nos. 35 and 36. Council Minutes dated 12 February 1942 record that the 'President reported that he had signed the contract for the purchase of No. 36 Lincoln's Inn Fields, that the site had been valued at £14,000 (£706,866)[9] and that the amount of the War Damage claim in respect of the building was £9,500 (£476,266)[9].'[34] In the Minutes of 14 October 1943, Council is recorded as having 'resolved that the premises of The College of Estate Management (No. 35 Lincoln's Inn Fields) be purchased for £65,000 (£3,152,548)[9] subject to contract and subject to agreement by the War Damage Commission to the assignment of the War Damage claim to this college.'[34] It was also resolved, 'That the President be authorised to negotiate for the purchase of No. 45 Lincoln's Inn Fields.'[34] Interestingly, the National Fire Service was given permission by RCS England to raise pigs, rabbits and chickens in the ruins of Nos. 35 to 38 until the end of the war (See Fig. 17).

Although eponymous lectures had been delivered since 1800, little effort had been made to teach postgraduate students. It was decided by Council and Sir Alfred Webb-Johnson, (1880-1958) elevated to the peerage in 1948, President of the Royal College of Surgeons of England (PRCS) from 1941 to 1949, to offer courses of lectures in anatomy, applied physiology and pathology to primary FRCS candidates from home and abroad beginning in 1946.[35]

These lectures adumbrated the formation of the Institute of Basic Medical Sciences (IBMS) in 1951.[35] Accommodation was problematic in the post-war period so it was resolved to construct a residential building on the bomb-site to the east that was to be substantial because of the far-sighted wartime property acquisitions and the generosity of Viscount Nuffield.

The automobile manufacturer and philanthropist, William Morris (1877-1963), elevated to the peerage in 1934 with the addition of a viscountcy in 1938, had promised £250,000 (£9.672 million)[9] as early as 1948.[35] Construction to a design by Alner W. Hall, MC, FRIBA, (1884-1971) architect to the college advised by

41

Sir Edward Maufe, RA, FRIBA (1882-1974), did not begin until 1951 because of post-war shortages of labour and materials.[36]

Work on the new building proceeded more or less in tandem with the rebuilding of RCS England that was formally reopened by Her Majesty Queen Elizabeth II (r. 1952-2022), accompanied by The Duke of Edinburgh (1921-2021), on 7 November, 1962.[36] The President's Lodge in the Nuffield College incorporated some fine seventeenth and eighteenth century architectural features salvaged from Nos. 44 and 45 that had been sold to the ICRF and were shortly to be demolished.[36] These were transferred to the new college building in 2021.

XVIII   The Nuffield College of Surgical Sciences 1957 to 2017

In 1976, I enrolled in a 12 week IBMS Primary Fellowship Course that was taught by Professors R.M.H. Mcminn (Applied Anatomy), Cyril Long (Biochemistry), J.L. Turk (Pathology), G.P. Lewis (Pharmacology) and D.E.M. Taylor (Physiology) with their readers and lecturers.[37]

The majority of postgraduate students on the course lived in the Nuffield (See Fig. 18). Common rooms on the first floor were spacious (See Fig. 19) and there were good-sized bedrooms on the upper floors with shared bathrooms and lavatories but the accommodation was spartan (See Fig. 20).[36]

Dinner in the Nuffield's impressive Webb-Johnson Hall panelled in chestnut and English oak, sometimes, became a special occasion! On 5 April, 1957, the new college was handed over to RCS England by Viscount Nuffield. It was then formally opened by Lt. Gen. Lord Freyberg, VC (1889-1963). In his speech, he stressed the importance of collegiate life and the opportunity it provided for postgraduate students to interact, informally, with their seniors (See Fig. 21).[38]

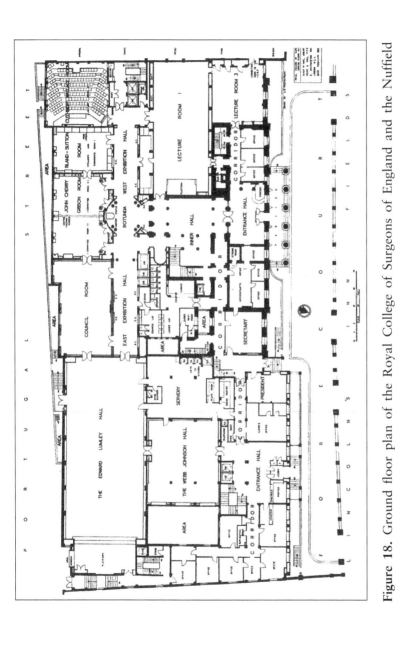

Figure 18. Ground floor plan of the Royal College of Surgeons of England and the Nuffield College of Surgical Sciences, 1957.
Alner W. Hall, MC, FRIBA, architect.
Courtesy of the Archives of the Royal College of Surgeons of England.

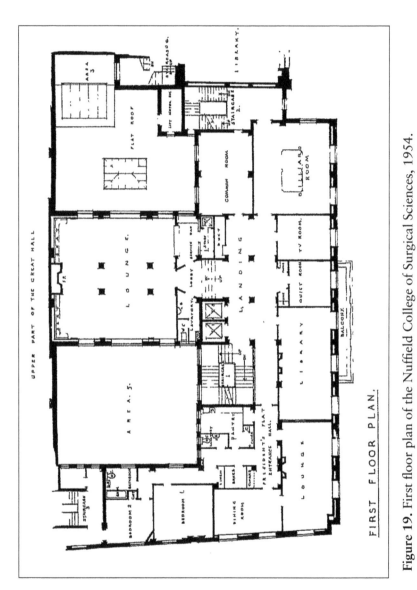

Figure 19. First floor plan of the Nuffield College of Surgical Sciences, 1954. Alner W. Hall, MC, FRIBA, architect. Courtesy of the Archives of the Royal College of Surgeons of England.

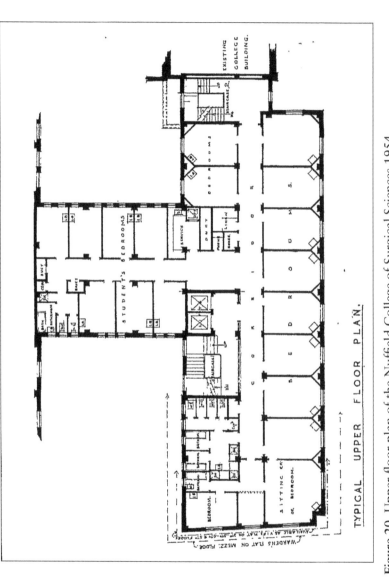

Figure 20. Upper floor plan of the Nuffield College of Surgical Sciences 1954. Alner W. Hall, MC, FRIBA, architect. Courtesy of the Archives of the Royal College of Surgeons of England.

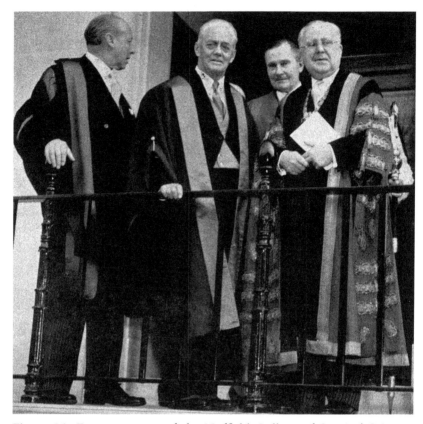

Figure 21. Front entrance of the Nuffield College of Surgical Sciences from a photograph in the *Annals of the Royal College of Surgeons of England* in May 1957. From left to right: Mr. Lawrence Abel, Vice-President, The Viscount Nuffield, Lt. Gen. The Lord Freyberg, VC, and Sir Harry Platt, PRCS at the opening ceremony on 5 April 1957. Courtesy of the Archives of the Royal College of Surgeons of England.

Our first encounter, at dinner, with a luminary of the college was with colorectal surgeon Alan Guyatt Parks (1920-1982) who had graduated from Oxford to become a wartime Rockefeller clinical student at the Johns Hopkins University School of Medicine in 1943. He was elected to Council in 1971 and knighted in 1977.[39] The hoary old complaint about the initialism 'RCS' standing for 'Retired College of Surgeons' was raised as a topic! Parks conceded that membership was concerned that Council consisted principally of London-based, elderly men and too many were retired full-time academics (his *bête noire*). From 1947, there had been grumbling about too many invited representatives of subspecialty associations, in addition to the elected 24! Parks also confirmed that deliberations of Council were secret and details of discussions were not entered in the minutes which, in any event, were not circulated to the members and fellows.

Sir Alan was elected PRCS in 1980 and there were high hopes of radical reform bringing about an open and transparent, elected Council, with realistic age and term limits, capable of representing the interests of practicing National Health Service (NHS) surgeons but, sadly, he died in office in November 1982 at the age of 62.[39] Sir Alan is still revered around the world as the most original and creative colorectal surgeon of the twentieth century.

In 2020, Timothy Lane in his final editorial as Editor-in-Chief of the *Annals of the Royal College of Surgeons of England* maintained that little has changed in the past 40 years.[38] 'Edicts and judgments passed down from Ivory Towers...' 'are rarely appreciated' and Council's failure to reflect the busy, diverse NHS workforce is a cause of alienation to this day.[40]

Australian-born Professor Raymond Jack Last, FRCS (1903-1993) was the author of the standard textbook '*Anatomy, Regional and Applied,*' first published in 1954, used by every primary fellowship candidate with new editions still in widespread use today. It was a welcome surprise to meet Professor Last at dinner in the Webb-Johnson Hall in May 1976.[41] He related that, after wartime service, he was appointed Anatomy Demonstrator and Curator at RCS England from 1946 to 1950 and Professor of Applied Anatomy from 1950 to 1970. In 1949, he became warden of the temporary accommodation for 20 postgraduate students in houses Nos. 44 and 45 to the west of the college and was the first warden of the Nuffield. Professor Last explained that he was living in retirement in Malta but always enjoyed a stopover in London on his way to Los Angeles where he continued as Visiting Professor of Anatomy at UCLA until 1988.[41]

There were some riotous evenings in the 'Lounge' on the first floor (See Fig. 19) when it was certain that the adjacent President's Lodge was unoccupied. PRCS at the time was the celebrated biliary and pancreatic surgeon, Sir Rodney Smith (1914-1998), later elevated to the peerage as Baron Smith of Marlow, who was sometimes in need of a bridge partner![42]

One evening, over dinner, Sir Rodney related an anecdote about Sir Anthony Eden's (1897-1977) bile duct injury sustained during an elective cholecystectomy on April 12, 1953, at Bart's. At a joint meeting of the American College of Surgeons and RCS England in London an American surgeon asked, 'can you tell me why your Prime Minister had to go to Boston to have his bile duct repaired?' An English surgeon replied, 'well, you chaps have had much more experience of bad biliary surgery than we have...'. Richard Cattell (1900-1964), Director of the Lahey Clinic then in Boston, and Rodney Smith were collaborators and friends.

In 1976, the historic position of Secretary of the College was held by a distinguished gentleman known as 'J-G', Ronald Stuart Johnson-Gilbert (1925-2003), who was justifiably proud of his direct ancestor, Dr. Samuel Johnson. There had been only five secretaries of the college from 1800 to 1962 when 'J-G' was appointed. He remained in office until 1988 serving with 10 presidents.[43] In 2011, in keeping with the times, the title was changed to CEO!

Sadly, the various makeover projects at the Nuffield, beginning in the late 1980s, after the demise of the IBMS, with 'hotel' accommodation and culminating in the so-called bicentenary project on the ground floor, proved to be something of an aesthetic and financial disaster.

XIX The Institute of Basic Medical Sciences 1951 to 1986

In 1986, the neo-Georgian Nuffield had become a potential white elephant after the phased withdrawal of funding for the IBMS by the British Postgraduate Medical Federation (BPMF), one of three postgraduate medical schools of the University of London, which was founded in 1945 and dissolved in 1996.[44] The others, at the time, were the London School of Hygiene and Tropical Medicine and the Royal Postgraduate Medical School (RPMS) based at the Hammersmith Hospital.

The Flowers' Report for the University of London in 1980 (*vide infra*) had stated that, 'the future of the Institute of Basic Medical Sciences does not lie with the university.'[45] RCS England created the 'Hunterian Institute of Surgical Education and Sciences' in an attempt to fund the six chairs in anatomy, biochemistry, pathology, pharmacology, physiology and ophthalmology that had been established by 1959.[34] By 1996, the crippling expense, despite the continuation of generous charitable donations and research grants to individuals, had enforced closures that began in 1992.[34]

XX The Faculties of Anaesthetists, Dental Surgery and General Dental Practice

There were three independent faculties associated with RCS England. The Faculty of Anaesthetists from 1948 with research facilities in the college that moved to the Nuffield in 1957; the Faculty of Dental Surgery (FDS) from 1947 with laboratories in the college and the Faculty of General Dental Practice (UK) (FGDP) from 1992 based in the Nuffield. The FGDP replaced the Anaesthetists who had formed their own college and departed in 1988. A royal charter was granted to the latter in 1992. The FGDP transferred to their new 'College of General Dentistry' on 1 July 2021. Members were invited to make a choice either to join the new college or to remain a member of RCS England through the FDS. Interestingly, a six member Dental Board consisting of three dentists and three surgeons had been authorised by a supplemental charter in 1859 to conduct a Licence in Dental Surgery (LDS) examination held for the first time on 13 March 1860.[46]

XXI Down House
The Buckston Browne Surgical Research Farm

Down House, home of Charles Darwin from 1842 to 1882, was purchased from Darwin's heirs by Sir George Buckston Browne, FRCS (1850-1945), a pioneer urologist, and presented to the British Association for the Advancement of Science in 1929.[47] It was donated to RCS England in 1953 when the endowment proved to be inadequate. In 1962, Sir Hedley Atkins (1905-1983), the first professor of surgery at Guy's Hospital Medical School (University of London) and a future PRCS, moved in with his wife, Gladys, and assumed the rôle of honorary curator. Down House was acquired from the college by English Heritage in 1996.[47]

The Buckston Browne Surgical Research Farm, adjacent to Down House, was endowed and presented to RCS England in 1931.[47] The aforementioned financial constraints in the 1980s led to drastic curtailment in activity after its heyday, including work on organ transplantation by Sir Roy Yorke Calne, FRCS, FRCP, FRS (born 1930), from the 1950s to the 1970s. This was the beginning of Cambridge-based Calne's collaboration with Professor Thomas Starzl (1926-2017) working at the University of Colorado in Denver from 1962 and successful liver transplantation. The building was sold in 1989 after a series of anti-vivisection protests.[34]

XXII The Royal Commission on Medical Education, 1968 (the Todd Report)

The Royal Commission, chaired by Nobel Laureate Lord Todd, PRS (1907-1997) a biochemist, produced its landmark report in 1968.[48] It was, itself, anticipated in some respects by the report on medical schools for the Ministry of Health in 1944 chaired by the banker Sir William Goodenough (1899-1951).[49] Reaction to Todd was mixed although the profession and the 20 member Royal

Commission endorsed the establishment of four new medical schools that began accepting students in Nottingham (1970), Southampton (1971), Leicester (1975), Swansea (2004) and a clinical school in Cambridge (1976).[48]

The Commission took the view that the undergraduate course in medicine should be primarily educational, 'it's object is to produce not a fully qualified doctor, but an educated man who will become fully qualified by postgraduate training.'[46] This would consist of general professional training marked with an exit qualification of membership of a college, higher specialist training, continuous assessment and an exit qualification of a college fellowship. These would be required for entry on to a new specialist register kept by the GMC. The abolition of all non-university qualifying examinations was also recommended.[48]

The significant advantages of 'close contact between the medical, natural, and social sciences at teaching and research level' stemming from undergraduate and postgraduate institutions, specialist hospitals and their research institutes becoming an integral part of multi-faculty colleges of universities were not immediately recognised except by doctors familiar with European and US universities.[48]

The conclusion that the 12 small medical schools associated with London's great, former voluntary hospitals would have to be paired prior to integration was not well-received by staff or students, past and present, mainly because of loyalties and tradition. London consultants were concerned about the 'United Hospitals Cup', the oldest rugby competition in the world, 'who are the boys going to play rugby against?'

The report was summarised by the *British Medical Journal* on 13 April 1968.[50] It was greeted with scepticism because it was understood to recommend the replacement of a system in use for more than a century that had resulted in British medicine and surgery becoming widely admired and highly respected at home and abroad. Doctors from overseas, including the US, competed for postgraduate attachments to world-renowned physicians and surgeons.[2] In fact, most of the proposed reforms of postgraduate training were not implemented until after the Calman Report in 1993 (vide infra).

XXIII   The Flowers Report 1980

In 1980, Lord Flowers, FRS (1924-2010), a physicist and Rector of the Imperial College of Science and Technology (ICL), was commissioned by the University of London to report on medical education in the city. Most of the 34 separate institutions in London whose futures were at stake correctly interpreted the Flowers' report to be another attempt to impose the Todd recommendations that were still being negotiated with no end in sight. The report was summarised by the British Medical Journal on 8 March 1980.[45]

In 1988, St. Mary's Hospital Medical School became the first to integrate with a university college forming the Imperial College of Science, Technology and Medicine.[51] Interestingly, Lord Flowers served as Vice-Chancellor of the University of London between 1985 and 1990 and his influence may have been decisive!

XXIV   The Tomlinson Inquiry 1992
versus the Todd Report

In 1992, an 'Inquiry into London's health services, medical education and research' for the Secretaries of State for Education and Health was made by Sir Bernard Tomlinson (1920-2017), a retired Professor of Pathology at Newcastle University, who had trained in London.[52] Todd, Flowers and Tomlinson followed similar reports every 10 years or so since 1890, emphasising the necessity of rationalising one aspect or another of health services in London. Their recommendations concerning the restructuring of medical education were out of kilter with each other but work in progress was based on the Todd Report. Today, Tomlinson is notorious for his proposal to reduce the overprovision of acute beds in London by closing Bart's, Charing Cross and the Middlesex Hospitals along with 10 smaller ones.[52]

The Middlesex Hospital did close in 2005 and its services were transferred to the new University College Hospital but Tomlinson's report was too controversial and was, effectively, ignored. 11 of the 12 historic teaching hospitals survived, including the Westminster resurrected, in 1993, as the Chelsea and Westminster on the site of the old St. Stephen's Hospital in the Fulham Road that incorporated St. Mary Abbot's, Westminster Children's and the West London Hospital. Charing Cross Hospital moved to a new building in the Fulham Palace Road in 1973 and the old hospital in Agar Street is now the Charing Cross Police Station!

University College Hospital was founded as the North London Hospital in 1834 and Scottish surgeon Robert Liston, FRCS, FRS (1794-1847) was appointed foundation Professor of Clinical Surgery in 1835.[53] He was one of the original 300 fellows elected on 11 December 1843 and had held the MRCS (Eng.) and the FRCS (Ed.) since 1818. The hospital was located opposite the main campus of UCL in Gower Street founded in 1828. In the days before anaesthesia surgeons vied with each other in speed and precision and their popularity was judged accordingly. Liston, known as 'the fastest knife in the West End' used to say that a cystolithotomy (removal of a stone from the bladder) should take only two or three minutes at most.[53] He was continually adding to his reputation by performing surgical feats which his colleagues declined to attempt such as his dexterous excision of a 44lb tumour of the scrotum which the patient used to carry around in a wheelbarrow. The most famous but probably apocryphal anecdote about Liston is of the occasion when he not only amputated a leg in 2½ minutes but also the fingers of his young assistant who was holding the patient and the coat tails of a spectator who died of 'fright!' The patient and the assistant later died of 'hospital gangrene' – the only recorded operation with a 300% mortality!

In fact, on 21 December 1846, Liston performed the first operation in Europe using ether as an anaesthetic to amputate the putrefying leg of a 36 year old man.[53] Liston commented, 'by God, gentlemen, this Yankee dodge beats mesmerism hollow' referring to American dental surgeon William Morton's (1819-1868) demonstration of ether anaesthesia earlier in the year at the Massachusetts General Hospital when a tumour of a man's neck was painlessly removed.[53] Some sources claim that Joseph Lister (vide supra) was present at the procedure but, as he didn't register as a medical student at UCL until 1848, and was reading for the compulsory premedical arts degree (he chose botany and classics), it seems unlikely but certainly possible.[53] Sadly, Liston died of a ruptured aortic aneurysm in December 1847 at the early age of 53.[53]

The famous 'Cruciform Building,' designed by Sir Alfred Waterhouse, PPRIBA, RA (1830-1905), that replaced the North London Hospital dates from 1905 and closed in 1995.[53] It was purchased by UCL, completely refurbished, and is now used by the medical faculty for biomedical research and as a teaching facility for bioscience and medical students.[53] The new hospital is north of Grafton Way with a main entrance in the Euston Road and was opened by The Queen in October 2005. Happily, the United Hospitals of London have been preserved along with their traditional sporting events and entertainments.

In 1983, Guy's and St Thomas's had been the first medical schools to merge.[54] They were followed by Charing Cross and the Westminster in 1984.[51] The Middlesex and University College merged in 1987.[53] St. George's Hospital was established in Lanesborough House, Hyde Park Corner in 1733.[55] Its medical school (SGUL), founded in 1834, is unique because it has been a constituent college of the University of London since the latter's foundation in 1836.[55] The hospital and medical school left one of the best addresses in London and moved to Tooting in 1980.[55] The original building was demolished and replaced by architect William Wilkins (1778-1839) between 1827 and 1834 and is now the Lanesborough Hotel.

Beginning in the mid-1990s, medical school mergers and university college integration, not precisely as envisaged by Todd or Flowers, were completed as follows (years in brackets refer to the year of foundation of the associated teaching hospital):

1. St. Bartholomew's (1123), The London (1740): Queen Mary College (QMUL) 1995.[56]
2. Guy's (1721), King's (1840), St. Thomas's (1173): King's College (KCL) 1998.[54]
3. Charing Cross (1818), St. Mary's (1845), Westminster (1719): Imperial College (ICL) 1997.[51] Imperial College became an independent university in 2007.
4. Royal Free (1828), Middlesex (1745), University College Hospital (1834): University College (UCL) 1998.[53]

The British Postgraduate Medical School (BPMS) founded in 1931 at the Hammersmith Hospital became part of the BPMF in 1947; 'Royal' (RPMS) and an independent school of the University of London in 1974; merged with the 'Institute of Obstetrics and Gynaecology' in 1986 and Imperial College School of Medicine in 1997.[51] The Lister Institute of Preventive Medicine was a postgraduate school of the University of London from 1905 to 1978 and the London School of Hygiene and Tropical Medicine from 1924 to date.[44] Please see Table 1 for membership, with dates, of the defunct British Postgraduate Medical Federation.

XXV   The National Health Service

The efficiency of the Emergency Hospital Service throughout the Second World War; the high standard of medical care provided to service personnel and, for the first time, a strong sense of social solidarity culminated in widespread support for the establishment of a National Health Service (NHS).

Table 1. Postgraduate Institutes, with dates, of the British Postgraduate Medical Federation, University of London, 1945 to 1996.

1. Basic Medical Sciences, Royal College of Surgeons of England 1951 to 1986.
2. British Postgraduate Medical School, Hammersmith Hospital 1947 to 1974.
3. Dental Surgery 1948 to 1992 (endowed by George Eastman of Eastman-Kodak).
4. Dermatology 1948 to 1990 (originally St. John's Institute of Dermatology founded in 1863).
5. Diseases of the Chest, Royal Brompton Hospital 1947 to 1972, Cardiothoracic Institute 1972 to 1988 and the National Heart and Lung Institute 1988 to 1995.
6. Cancer Research, Royal Marsden Hospital from 1947. Associate college of the University of London from 1995 and a constituent college from 2003.
7. Cardiology, National Heart Hospital from 1947, formed the Cardiothoracic Institute at the Brompton in 1972.
8. Child Health, Hospital for Sick Children, Great Ormond Street 1948 to 1995.
9. Laryngology and Otology, Royal National Throat, Nose and Ear Hospital 1947 to 1988.
10. Neurology, National Hospital for Neurology and Neurosurgery 1950 to 1995.
11. Obstetrics and Gynaecology, Hammersmith Hospital, 1948 to 1986. Royal Postgraduate Medical School 1986 to 1997.
12. Ophthalmology, Moorfields Eye Hospital 1948 to 1995.
13. Orthopaedics, Royal National Orthopaedic Hospital 1947 to 1988.
14. Psychiatry, Maudsley and Bethlem Royal Hospitals 1948 to 1995.
15. Urology, St. Peter's Hospital for Stone 1954 to 1988.

On 5 July 1948, the appointed day, all UK hospitals were nationalised and subsumed by the new National Health Service.[57] There were 1,143 voluntary hospitals with about 90,000 beds and 1,545 municipal hospitals, most of which had evolved from the old Poor Law workhouse infirmaries, with about 390,000 beds in total.[57] At least, 190,000 of these were used for the treatment of mental illness and mental handicap.[57]

Acute care practice in the former voluntary hospitals, and later in the municipal ones, continued to be organised on the old 'firm' system consisting of two consultants (previously honorary), one long-serving and highly experienced senior registrar (SR), two registrars and two house surgeons.[2] The admitting firm managed all their own emergencies from admission to discharge thereby guaranteeing that vital ingredient for the best possible outcome for the patient - continuity of care.[2]

Surgical training remained an overarching apprenticeship and was the responsibility of RCS England.[2] The process of enhancing medical scientific knowledge included college, association and society meetings; lectures and courses; weekly clinicopathological conferences; weekly journal clubs initiated by Professor William Osler (1849-1919) in 1875 whilst at McGill; higher degrees; research (often in the US) and publication.[2]

Aneurin (Nye) Bevan (1897-1960), Labour Minister of Health from 1945 to 1951, introduced the National Health Service Act in 1946. He wanted to have a prestigious, high quality service that he believed could not be achieved without the support of hospital consultants – the country's 'top doctors.'[58] Therefore, against his better judgment, he made major concessions to the self-interested views of the three medical royal colleges in London (physicians, surgeons, obstetricians and gynaecologists).[58] Consultants were to be 'paid for work that they had previously done for nothing;' to have loosely defined NHS sessions; the right to private practice in NHS and private hospitals; 'the secret disposal of Treasury funds' (distinction awards) to those thought more meritorious by their college presents and the 'lion's share' of teaching hospital endowments for research.[59]

The matter was settled over dinner at Prunier's restaurant in St. James's Street between the Minister and Winston Churchill's personal physician, Lord Moran (1882-1977), President of the Royal College of Physicians.[58] Whilst Bevan and Moran were enjoying dinner, the 'negotiating committee under the aegis of the British Medical Association was awaiting a summons to Whitehall.'[58] When Bevan was asked, years later, how he had managed to persuade hospital consultants to support the creation of the National Health Service he replied, 'I stuffed their mouths with gold.'[59] This remark was authenticated by Webster (1991) and was probably made in late 1955 or early 1956.[60] Teaching hospital consultants with many commitments, including large private practices and limited NHS sessions, relied on the support of their junior staff all of whom were in training although the emphasis was clearly on the service component.

XXVI   The Doctors' Mess

The Doctors' Mess was a legacy of the voluntary hospital movement and run like an Officers' Mess. They were a privilege that NHS administrators were obsessed with eliminating, ostensibly on grounds of economy but, more likely, in the interests of egalitarianism. In the armed forces there was a daily messing charge, but expenses not covered by NHS hospitals, such as provisioning and bar bills, were defrayed by contributing the fees paid for signing cremation forms irreverently known as 'ash cash.'

Junior medical staff enjoyed mess life (not to mention mess parties and other diversions) because most were working 120 hours per week acquiring the breadth and depth of experience necessary for independent practice. The European Working Time Directive (EWTD) did not exist! Nevertheless, by the mid-1990s, most messes had been closed by the lay administration that then turned its attention to emasculating the medical profession by eradicating the long-established 'consultant is king' culture with the support, no doubt, of left wing governments!

XXVII   The Calman Report 1993

Sir Kenneth Calman (born 1941), Chief Medical Officer (CMO) for England produced a report for the government in 1993 entitled, 'Hospital Doctors: Training for the Future: the Report of the Working Group on Specialist Medical Training.'[61] The EU Commission had declared that UK specialist training was 'illegal' because there were no exit examinations or other definable end point and Calman's purpose was to comply with EU directives on harmonisation that had been ignored by the UK for years.[2] His training paradigm, adumbrated by the Todd and Flowers Reports, was to be structured and, unlike its predecessor, time-limited.[2] Historic job titles were to be abolished and the emphasis was to be on education rather than service. Progression would be based on objectively assessed competence rather than time served and a consultant's opinion.[2]

The government legalised Calman's proposals by means of a Statutory Instrument (SI) entitled the 'European Specialist Medical Qualifications Order, 1995' effective from 12 January 1996, which established the Specialist Training Authority (STA) of the medical royal colleges.[2] A second SI in 2005 abolished the STA and formed the independent Postgraduate Medical Education and Training Board (PMETB) that was merged with the GMC by yet another SI in 2010.[2] Thus, the GMC assumed ultimate responsibility for specialist training formerly the remit of the medical royal colleges.[2] Nevertheless, the 23 medical royal colleges and faculties in the UK and Ireland that comprise the Academy of Medical Royal Colleges, founded in 1974, all claim to be active in providing educational activities of various kinds for specialists-in-training and also in the monitoring of standards.[62]

'Intercollegiate' refers to the three UK surgical royal colleges, England, Edinburgh, and Glasgow along with the Royal College of Surgeons in Ireland. In January 2004, the new Intercollegiate MRCS replaced the old-style final FRCS as an assessment of suitability for higher surgical training (HST).[8] It was taken after the preregistration year and up to five years as a senior house officer (SHO) undertaking vocational posts, fellowships, research (often overseas) or higher degrees.[62]

Specialty FRCS diplomas were not introduced until after the implementation of Calman although the college had awarded a final FRCS diploma in ophthalmology (OPHTH) from 1921 and otorhinolaryngology (ORL) from 1947.[35] Since 1988, the Royal College of Ophthalmologists has conducted its own examinations and awards the MRCOphth and the FRCOphth. The MRCS and FRCS examinations are now administered by the 'Joint Committee on Intercollegiate Examinations' (JCIE) and not by the individual colleges as they were prior to the first Intercollegiate MRCS examination in January 2004. FRCS exit examinations in the following subspecialties are available: cardiothoracic surgery, general surgery, neurosurgery, oral and maxillofacial surgery, otolaryngology, paediatric surgery, plastic surgery, trauma and orthopaedic surgery, urology and vascular surgery. Successful candidates are eligible for election to the fellowship of any one of the four surgical royal colleges and use of its postnominal.

The Joint Surgical Colleges' Fellowship Examinations (JSCFE) are offered to international surgeons-in-training and organised by the JSCFE Committee in cardiothoracic surgery, general surgery, neurosurgery, trauma and orthopaedic surgery and urology. Passing the examination confers eligibility for election as a fellow to one of the four colleges and use of its postnominal.

The old-style FRCS which had survived for 161 years from 1843 to 2004 metamorphosed into its new rôle as an Intercollegiate exit examination at the conclusion of six years' HST in a chosen specialty. It was required, with a Certificate of Completion of Specialist Training (CCST) for entry on to the GMC's new specialist register.[6] These were mandatory requirements for a consultant appointment in the NHS achieved, on average, 12 years after qualification.[62] From 1998, opportunities for trainees to gain experience were significantly reduced by the EWTD that was fully implemented by 2009 and replaced by Working Time Regulations (WTR) after Brexit.[63]

Interestingly, a group of lobbyists, led by the venerable Professor Harold Ellis, Emeritus Professor of Surgery at Westminster Hospital Medical School (University of London), has been advocating for years for the return of the surgical firm in order to re-establish continuity of care that was disrupted by the EWTD but may be equally frustrated by the WTR!

XXVIII   Modernising Medical Careers 2005

A report, in 2002, by Calman's successor, Sir Liam Donaldson (born 1949) entitled '*Unfinished Business*' was intended to address long-standing problems with the senior house officer (SHO) grade.[62] By 2005, it had expanded into '*Modernising Medical Careers*' (MMC) that modified most levels of postgraduate training, sometimes constructively, and the widely criticised '*Medical Training Application Service*' (MTAS).[62] MMC introduced two foundation years of which the first year was the preregistration internship. Subsequently, two years' core surgical training (CST) and six years' HST required two competitive applications. However, Donaldson had instituted 'run-through' training (combining CST and HST) and successful candidates applied only once.[62] Donaldson also replaced Calman's specialist registrars (SpR) with specialty registrars (StR - followed by a number indicating the year of training), his CCST with a Certificate of Completion of Training (CCT) and introduced 'workplace-based assessment' (WBA).[62]

61

MTAS created such chaos that applications had to revert to a local process determined by regional deaneries and the colleges.[62] By 2011, CST had been decoupled from HST in most surgical specialties except neuro, cardiothoracic and maxillofacial surgery. Run-throughs eventually became popular with trainees and pilot studies that include general surgery were resumed in August 2018.[64] After MMC, most surgical trainees are awarded a CCT approximately 10 years after qualification but longer if 'time-out' has been requested to undertake research or proceed to a higher degree. However, HST does include a requirement to publish three peer-reviewed research papers and to make three presentations to learned societies.[2]

Interested institutions continued to produce proposals in the form of reports such as *'Aspiring to Excellence'* (2007); *'Foundation for Excellence'* (2010); *'Future Hospital: caring for medical patients'* (2013) and the *'Shape of Training'* (2013).[62] Discussions are still ongoing regarding the place of post-CCT fellowship training and credentialing in specialty areas of particular complexity that are undertaken by 80 per cent of general surgeons in the US.[2]

XXIX Intercollegiate Surgical Curriculum Programme (ISCP)

Since 2007, curricula in 10 surgical specialties are formulated by the ISCP.[65] These are general, cardiothoracic, neuro, oral and maxillofacial, otorhinolaryngology, paediatric, plastic, trauma and orthopaedic, urology and (more recently) vascular surgery.[65] Since the aforementioned merger with the PMETB in 2010, the ISCP is responsible to the GMC.[8] Surgical competency is judged by 'direct observation of procedural skills' (DOPS) and 'procedure based assessment' (PBA). Important components of assessment are the 'Annual Review of Competence Progression' (ARCP), the 'Multiple Consultant Report' (MCR) at the middle and end of each placement and the 'Assigned Educational Supervisor' (AES) report at the end of the placement.[65] Since 2012, the Calman/ MMC/ISCP system of specialist training has been administered by 'Health Education England' (HEE) which has responsibility for the education and training of all NHS healthcare professionals and is to merge with NHS England probably in 2023. Medical specialist training now operates through four national directors and 13 'Local Education and Training Boards' (LETBs) that replaced the old postgraduate deaneries but often not in the same geographical locations.[62]

Each LETB has created a 'School of Surgery' that provides structure for 'corporate' and financial governance and the coordination of educational, organisational and quality management activities of surgical training programmes.[62] They ensure the use of ISCP curricula and assessment methods and provide any necessary training for surgeon educators.[62] A challenge is likely to be the provision of sophisticated (and expensive) virtual reality and robotic simulation equipment with the necessary trained staff. Since the demise of the 'see one, do one, teach one' paradigm, because of the advent of high technology surgery in the 1990s, it is important to steepen the learning curve on patients - in the mathematical rather than the colloquial sense – or perhaps eliminate it altogether.

XXX   The New Breed of Surgeons

In any event, a revolution in surgical training, qualification and practice began in the mid-1990s leaving many senior fellows in the rear-view mirror. The influence of Todd, Calman and Donaldson was profound along with the aforementioned advances in the medical sciences, engineering and high technology.[2] Many older general surgeons learned basic laparoscopy (hernias and gallbladders) from the early-1990s, but relatively few mastered the increasingly sophisticated techniques that have enabled surgical treatment of a continuously expanding spectrum of disease.[2] However, more than 50 RCTs so far have shown that procedures using robotic technology such as the 'da Vinci Surgical

System' are expensive and prolonged with outcomes that are no better, and sometimes worse, than standard video-assisted minimally invasive or open surgery. Data continues to be collected but the jury is still out *(vide infra)*![66]

It remains to be seen whether the new breed of surgeons is adequately serving the needs of surgical patients, producing the best possible outcomes and sustaining the high international reputation for surgical practice and innovation earned by their predecessors.[2] If so, the 'oldies' can only doff their hats to their successors and look forward to the approaching era of artificial intelligence (AI) in healthcare. AI was predicted by Alan Turing (1912-1954) the mathematician and pioneer of computer science, in 1950, with his paper on the 'Turing Test.'[67] AI in healthcare may evolve significantly in the next few decades but, currently its rôle is uncertain.[68]

XXXI Surgical Volume and Outcomes

Studies of the relationship between the volume of complex surgical procedures and outcomes began in 1979 at Stanford and the University of California San Francisco (UCSF) and may be relevant to current surgical practice.[69] Data, supported by common sense, are confirming that high-volume surgeons working in high-volume institutions achieve the best outcomes in bariatric, cardiac, oncological, transplantation and vascular surgery.[70] Superior outcomes are also seen in higher risk patients in most surgical specialties undergoing complex surgery in busy tertiary referral centers, either regional or national, which specialise in specific open, laparoscopic and robotically assisted procedures.[70] Lack of experience at secondary care level may account for disappointing outcomes particularly when using the £2 million 'da Vinci Surgical System' that does not, at present, provide haptic feedback. Promising tactile sensing technologies are under development and, hopefully, will become commercially available in the near future.

'Failure to rescue' patients with complications may be a feature of secondary care institutions that lack sufficient volumes of such patients and multidisciplinary teams to care for them. Germany has had minimum number requirements for most major surgery for 17 years and some state health departments in the US may follow suit.[70] There may be implications for general surgeons; part-time surgeons; those who take long breaks to have or raise a family; surgeons who find themselves on the receiving end and for the organisation of surgical care. The UK has published the outcomes of named consultants within most specialties since 2013 which seems to have resulted in some surgeons 'gaming' the data and also refusing to operate on high risk patients! Data relating to facilities are not provided.

The NHS Long Term Plan, 2019 does not address the issue specifically but confirms that treatment of rare or complex conditions will continue to be provided.[71] NHS England spent £17.2 billion in 2018-19 on 'specialised services' sometimes in modernised, historic hospitals that have provided tertiary care for 150 years and have the ability to recruit teams of staff with appropriate expertise. Others are located in brand-new, purpose-built and equipped institutions, mostly in Central London, and usually not far from their site of origin.[71] Please see Table 2 for a summary of restructuring, with dates, of London's multidisciplinary and/or principally surgical specialist (tertiary referral) hospitals and research institutes. The specialist hospitals remain closely associated with their former research institutes, sometimes physically, and both are now an integral part of a university college. Happily, the necessity of improving NHS screening services is finally acknowledged with specific proposals.[72]

Table 2. Summary of the restructuring, with dates, of London's multidisciplinary and specialist surgical (tertiary referral) hospitals and research institutes.

Tertiary Referral Hospital	Date	Research Institute	University Affiliation	Date
Royal Brompton	1842	Institute of Diseases of the Chest 1947.	UoL	1947
		Cardiothoracic Institute 1972	UoL	1972
		National Heart and Lung Institute formed in 1995.	ICL	1995
Harefield merged with the Brompton in 1998	1915	Brompton and Harefield are administered by Guy's and St. Thomas' NHS Foundation Trust since 2021.	ICL	1995
National Heart (Closed 1991)	1857	Institute of Cardiology from 1947 merged with the Cardiothoracic Institute at the Brompton in 1972.	UoL	1947
Royal Marsden	1851	Institute of Cancer Research 1909. ULC 1927-47	ULC	2003
St. Mark's Rectum & Colon (Northwick Park from 1995)	1835	St. Mark's Academic Institute 1995. Previously self-funded with ICRF support from 1986.	ICL	1995
Sick Children (GOS)	1852	Institute of Child Health 1946.	UCL	1996

RN Throat, Nose and Ear (Closed 2019)	1874	Institute of Laryngology and Otology 1947.	UCL	1988
		Royal National ENT and Eastman Dental Hospital	UCL	2019
NH for Neurology and Neurosurgery	1859	Institute of Neurology 1950. New facilities open in 2024 with a 'Dementia Unit' supported by the MRC.	UCL	1997
Moorfields Eye	1805	Institute of Ophthalmology 1948.	UCL	1995
Hammersmith	1902	Institute of Obstetrics and Gynaecology 1948 -1997	ICL	1997
RN Orthopaedic Stanmore	1840	Institute of Orthopaedics founded in 1944 by the British Orthopaedic Association.	UCL	1988
St Peter's for Stone, ('the three Ps' St Peter's, St Paul's and St Philip's plus the Shaftesbury). Moved to the Middlesex in 1992	1860	Institute of Urology 1954 Tertiary care beds provided by University College London Hospitals NHS Foundation Trust. The Middlesex Hospital closed in 2005 and its services moved to the new University College Hospital.	UCL	1988

Glossary: GOS - Great Ormond Street; ICL - Imperial College London; MRC - Medical Research Council; NH - National Hospital; RN - Royal National; UCL - University College London; UoL - University of London; ULC - constituent college of the University of London.

XXXII   The Magic Bullet

The medical profession has been waiting patiently for a 'magic bullet'[73] since physicist Francis Crick (1916-2004) and biologist James Watson (born 1928) working at the Cavendish Laboratory, Cambridge and X-ray crystallographer (and physical chemist) Rosalind Franklin (1920-1958) at KCL discovered DNA's double-helix in 1953. Crick, Watson and Maurice Wilkins (1916-2004), also an X-ray crystallographer and a physicist at KCL, shared the 1962 Nobel Prize in Physiology or Medicine.[74]

Dr. Franklin's calculations and her famous 'photo 51,' unbeknownst to her, were shared by Wilkins with Crick and Watson who immediately understood and capitalised on their significance. Regrettably, her vital contribution was not credited until long after her untimely death from ovarian cancer and the facts of the matter are still in dispute half a century later![75]

Fortunately, from the year 2000, breakthroughs in molecular biology and biotechnology have been mind-boggling. Currently, BioNTech (Mainz, Germany) and 'ModeRNA' (Cambridge, MA, US) are working on mRNA treatments in the following areas: auto-immune, cardiovascular, infectious and rare diseases, personalised cancer vaccines and immuno-oncology. Moderna has 14 clinical trials underway reporting encouraging preliminary data. Perhaps, the spectrum of disease currently being treated surgically will begin to contract.

XXXIII   The Revolution in Surgical Practice after the Second World War

The aforementioned advances after the Second World War in the medical sciences, engineering, high technology and surgical techniques resulted in a dramatic expansion of surgically treatable disease. Some examples are organ transplantation that began with the first human kidney transplant in 1954 by Nobel Laureate Joseph Murray (1919-2021) at the Peter Bent Brigham Hospital in Boston, MA. The first successful liver transplant was performed in 1967 by Thomas Starzl (1926-2017) then Professor of Surgery at the University of Colorado in Denver.

Professor Sir Roy Calne (born 1930) started the transplantation programme at the University of Cambridge in 1965 and performed the first liver transplant in the UK (and Europe) in 1968. His remarkable thirty-year partnership with hepatologist Roger Williams (1931-2020), Director of the Liver Unit at King's College Hospital, London began in 1966. There was also a trans-Atlantic alliance with Professor Starzl's unit in Denver that continued after Starzl's move to the University of Pittsburgh in 1981. Professor Calne performed the world's first liver, heart and lung transplant with Professor John Wallwork (born 1946) in 1987 at Papworth Hospital, Cambridge; the first intestinal transplant in the UK in 1992 and the first successful combined stomach, intestine, pancreas, liver and kidney cluster transplant in 1994. Throughout his career, Professor Calne played a major rôle in the development of immunosuppressants (chemotherapeutic anti-rejection medication).

Cardiopulmonary bypass was pioneered by surgeon John Gibbon (1903-1973) at the Jefferson Hospital in Philadelphia which was used for the first time in 1953 and underwent rapid development, initially, by groups at the Mayo Clinic led by surgeon John Kirklin (1917-2004) and at the University of Minnesota led by surgeon C. Walton Lillehei (1918-1999) who is often referred to as 'the father of open heart surgery.' A brand-new healthcare professional called a 'cardiovascular perfusionist' rapidly became indispensable. Coronary artery bypass grafting, valve replacement, congenital defect correction and transplantation were to become standard procedures. The first successful internal mammary-coronary artery bypass graft using a short tantalum cannula was performed by Robert Goetz (1910-2000) at the Bronx Municipal Hospital in New York in 1960 and the first saphenous vein graft by Rene Favaloro (1923-2000) at the Cleveland Clinic in 1967. Favaloro reported a successful series of 150 patients one year later. The first successful heart transplant was performed by Christiaan Barnard (1922-2001) in Cape Town, South Africa in 1967.

In the UK, the first successful heart transplant was performed by Sir Terence English (born 1932) at Papworth Hospital but not until August 1979. It was delayed because the Chief Medical Officer for England, Sir George Godber (1908-2009) decided that more research was needed into the management of rejection and imposed a moratorium in 1973. His decision was based on poor outcomes by Donald Ross (1922-2014) at the National Heart Hospital from 1968 and also by surgeons in Europe and the US.

Flexible endoscopes were developed by gastroenterologist Basil Hirschowitz (1925-2013) and his team at the University of Michigan and introduced in 1957 facilitating the performance of all endoscopies but, particularly, upper and lower gastrointestinal (GI) examinations that were required for screening, diagnosis and therapy. Endoscopic Retrograde Cholangiopancreatography (ERCP) was accomplished for the first time in 1968 by William McCune (1909-1998) at George Washington University Hospital in DC where he was Professor of Clinical Surgery for 35 years!

Sir John Charnley (1911-1982) performed the first low frictional torque total hip arthroplasty in 1962 at Wrightington Hospital in Lancashire. He designed the prosthesis himself which, subsequently, required a change of bearing surface material, Also at Wrightington, on a 'travelling hip arthroplasty fellowship' Canadian surgeon, Frank Gunston (1933-2016), designed and implanted the first knee prosthesis in 1971 which became known as the 'Gunston polycentric knee arthroplasty.'

Sonography has a long history but its use for diagnosis in clinical practice dates from a classic paper in *The Lancet* published on 7 June 1958 by Ian Donald (1910-1987), Regius Professor of Midwifery at the University of Glasgow, his registrar, John

MacVicar (1927-2011) and electrical engineer Thomas Brown (1933-2018).[76] John MacVicar was appointed foundation Professor of Obstetrics and Gynaecology at the University of Leicester Medical School in 1975.

Computerised Axial Tomography (CAT) uses X-rays (ionising radiation) and was introduced into clinical practice in 1972 by electrical engineer Sir Godfrey Hounsfield (1919-2004), working at 'Electric and Musical Industries' (EMI) that became known as the EMI scanner. Hounsfield shared the Nobel Prize in Physiology or Medicine in 1979 with American physicist Allan Cormack (1924-1988) who had published on the theory of CAT in the *Journal of Applied Physics* in 1963 and 1964. Cormack and Hounsfield did not meet until the Nobel ceremony and Hounsfield was unaware of Cormack's publications. CAT was described as the greatest advance in imaging since German engineer and physicist Wilhelm Röntgen (1845-1923) discovered X-rays almost by accident in 1895 and won the first Nobel Prize in Physics in 1901.

MRI is based on the phenomenon of nuclear magnetic resonance (NMR) first described in 1938 by physicist Isidor Rabi (1898-1988) working at Columbia University for which he was awarded the Nobel Prize in Physics in 1944. The 1952 prize was shared by physicists Edward Purcell (1912-1997) at Harvard and Felix Bloch (1905-1983) at Stanford for the development of NMR technology. The American physical chemist Paul Lauterbur (1929-2007) at Stony Brook University and physicist Sir Peter Mansfield (1933-2017) at Nottingham University, working independently, transformed NMR from a spectroscopic laboratory discipline into a clinical imaging technology known as Magnetic Resonance Imaging (MRI) that was introduced in 1977. Lauterbur and Mansfield shared the Nobel Prize in Physiology or Medicine in 2003. MRI surpasses CAT because it provides greater detail without the risks of ionising radiation and is particularly useful for the diagnosis of brain and spinal cord lesions.

German surgeon Erich Mühe's (1938-2005) series of 97 laparoscopic cholecystectomies, using instruments of his own design, began with the first laparoscopic cholecystectomy (LC) in history on 12 September 1985 and the series was completed in early 1987. Mühe's pioneering work at his hospital in Böblingen, 12 miles from Stuttgart, initiated the exciting era of minimally invasive surgery and revolutionised surgical practice around the world. The technique would be facilitated by the development, from 1982, of the solid state video camera and high resolution TV screens. In April 1986, the Congress of the German Society of Surgery (DGCH) in Munich reacted to Mühe's presentation with derisive comments such as 'Mickey Mouse surgery' and 'small brain, small incision.' His remarkable achievement was not embraced by the DGCH until 1992 when it was evident that LC was becoming a gold standard. Furthermore, the Society of American Gastrointestinal and Endoscopic Surgeons (SAGES) did not recognise Mühe as the originator of the technique until 1999 because of a competing claim by French surgeon Philippe Mouret (1938-2008) who had performed his first LC in Lyon on 17 March 1987 which, in fact, was the first to be video-assisted.

American physician Avedis Donabedian (1919-2000), working at the University of Michigan from 1961, became known as the 'father of quality assurance' after the publication of his lengthy paper in *The Milbank Memorial Fund Quarterly* in 1966 entitled *'Evaluating the Quality of Medical Care.'* Subsequently, he summarised his work in three volumes entitled *'Explorations in Quality Assessment and Monitoring'* published between 1980 and 1985.[77]

Last, but by no means least, Scottish physician Archibald (A. L.) Cochrane (1909-1988), was Director of the Medical Research Council's (MRC) Epidemiology Unit in Cardiff, South Wales, from 1960. He designed and conducted randomised controlled trials (RCTs) as described in his landmark book entitled *'Effectiveness and Efficiency: Random Reflections on Health Services (The Rock Carling Fellowship 1971)'* published in 1972.[78] RCTs play a major role in the practise of evidence-based medicine as defined by the 'Agency for Healthcare Research and Quality' (AHRQ), an agency of the US Department of Health and Human Services. 'Evidence-based medicine is an interdisciplinary approach which uses techniques from science, engineering, biostatistics and epidemiology, such as meta-analysis, decision analysis, risk-benefit analysis, and randomised controlled trials.' Johns Hopkins Division of General Internal Medicine writes, 'that the practice of evidence-based medicine uses systematic reviews of the medical literature to evaluate the best evidence on specific clinical topics. This evidence is used by practitioners to select treatment options for specific cases based on the best research, patient preferences and individual patient characteristics.'

XXXIV   RCS England in the Twenty-first Century

It is clear that, for centuries, RCS England and its predecessors were under the continuous control of distinguished surgeons at the end of their careers. The governing gerontocracies they formed were constituted to serve their own interests with the connivance of elderly cronies in high places. Arcane, archaic and undemocratic practices inherited from the livery companies and attacked 200 years ago by Thomas Wakley, in person and in *The Lancet*, continue to this day.

The college is still widely regarded by cynics as a congenial London club for elderly Council members who enjoy prancing around in scarlet and gold attending dinners and ceremonies of various kinds. Honorary fellowships are distributed to the 'great and good' in expectation of continuing the charitable donations that are believed by many to keep the gravy train running!

This narrative mentions some examples of the unintended consequences of undemocratic and unwise decisions based, sometimes, on unwillingness to embrace the relentless advance of medical science. In fact, the NHS encourages autocratic tendencies because it was, from the beginning, a highly centralised and undemocratic institution with appointed members on all its boards. 'Aneurin Bevan, its founder, came to regret this defect admitting that election is a better principle than selection.'[79]

The elected, 24 member Council decreed by the royal charter of 1843 survived until 1947 when Council, not unreasonably, decided that subspecialties without an elected member should be represented by invitation. In 1988, nine specialist associations and 'Accident and Emergency' were empowered to select a representative resulting in over-representation of several specialties that continues to this day. Lack of interest is suggested by the fact that only about one-third of eligible voters bothered to cast a ballot in Council elections and only one-third of subspecialists in the 'selection' of association appointees!

In 2015 appointees, seen by some as unworthy of a Council seat, became full members thereby exacerbating the alienation of the college membership whose opinion that this was a violation of democratic principle was, clearly, of no consequence! Council now comprises, at least, 36 full members whereas a cabinet of 22 ministers governs the UK!

Council's decision-making is minuted but not circulated to members and fellows; deliberations remain unrecorded and online referenda are rarely used. It is hard to conceive that the future of such a venerable institution may be in doubt except as a repository for the history of surgery and its artefacts. The elitist 'ivory-tower' in Lincoln's Inn Fields has always seemed unaware of the need for an open, transparent and elected Council accurately reflecting the busy, diverse workforce of practising surgeons throughout England and Wales.

The majority of young surgeons live and work outside London and regard the college as an irrelevance, albeit an expensive one. It is trainees and practising NHS surgeons who provide the bulk of the funding but only to continue using its postnominals if they have opted for election to the English fellowship![27] They have no other connection with the college since the introduction of HEE in 2012 and its proposed merger with NHS England in 2023! Even the college journals are occasionally subject to scoffing comments by those who remember the meticulous editing of Sir Cecil Wakeley, Tony Rains, Jerry Kirk, Sir Barry Jackson, John Lumley, Irving Taylor and Colin Johnson.

Courageously, in the summer of 2020, Professor Neil Mortensen the newly elected President of the Royal College of Surgeons of England invited Baroness Helena Kennedy, QC to produce a *'Diversity and Inclusion Review'* that was published on 18 March 2021. Sadly, the report concluded that the college and the profession are systemically 'sexist, racist and homophobic.'[80] The Baroness is very experienced in these matters and it was distressing to read that the problem of white male surgeons practising misogyny, sexual harassment, instinctive racism, implicit bias and homophobia is widespread![79]

In the US, the problem of racism is widely regarded as unsolvable, at least in the short term, but sexual harassment has become a dangerous pastime due to the powerful '#Me Too' movement. In the UK, ethnic minority surgeons have won, and continue to win, every 'glittering prize' available to successful surgeons. For example, Gold Coast/Ghanaian-born general surgeon Lord (Bernard) Ribeiro, PPRCS (born 1944) and Egyptian-born cardiac surgeon Professor Sir Magdi Yacoub OM, FRCS, FRS, Lister Medal 2015 (born 1935) were knighted, and the former was elevated to the peerage.

Many highly respected female surgeons are elected to Council and have been for 30 years. For example, Consultant Paediatric Surgeon, Leela Kapila, OBE, FRCS (born to an Indian family in 1937 on the family estate in Burma now Myanmar) was elected to Council in 1992 and to the Senior-Vice-Presidency in 2003. Throughout a long career in surgery at home and overseas, I have had the pleasure and privilege of working with women and surgeons of both sexes from ethnic minorities including

Miss Kapila. My colleagues and I were unaware of either racial discrimination or sexual harassment probably because of our naïveté! There was, and perhaps still is, an attitude that colleagues whatever their sex or ethnicity were either 'nice or nasty' and usually the diagnosis was not difficult!

The *Kennedy Review* implies that there is a considerable number of bigots in surgical practice without insight into the atavism of instinct and culture from which they suffer. The college's *'Diversity, Equity and Inclusion Action Plan'* (DEI) dated 16 September 2021 is a credit to its authors under the aegis of Professor Neil Mortensen, but challenging and likely to be plagued by disappointment and setbacks.[81] Even 'major efforts to reduce implicit bias formed over a lifetime show that any positive effects tend to wear off after a few hours or days.'[82] Much will depend on the mindset of surgeons which is unlikely to differ from the highly educated staff employed by major corporations who have been studied in detail by social scientists for many years.[82]

The Equality Act 2010 consolidated previous legislation and protects from direct and indirect discrimination, harassment and victimisation. The Act applies to discrimination based on age, race, sex, gender reassignment, disability, religion or belief, sexual orientation, marriage or civil partnership, pregnancy and motherhood. In the healthcare setting legal protection is rarely invoked despite being the only course of action likely to be effective probably for fear of exacerbating extant ill-feeling. Affirmative action remains illegal in the UK (and the EU) because it violates the principle of equal treatment.

So far, it appears that Professor Neil Mortensen may be our long awaited reformist president and, certainly, changes to the composition of Council and to its arcane and archaic practices would be warmly welcomed. If successfully implemented, along with the *DEI Action Plan,* the college could be transformed into a relevant institution supported by its members and fit to lead the body of surgeons into the future.

References

1. Jessie Dobson and Robert Milnes Walker, *A History of the Barbers and Barbet-Surgeons' Companies of London* (Oxford: Blackwell Scientific, 1979): xvii-xix, 9, 24.

2. John S, Bolwell, 'Surgical practice, then and now: the 5th to the 21st Century,' *Bulletin of the Royal College of Surgeons of England* 102, no. 3 (March 2020): 94-101, https://doi.org/10.1308/rcsbull.2020.94 (Accessed December 2021).

3. John McNee, 'Barber-Surgeons in Great Britain and Ireland (Thomas Vicary Lecture 30 October 1958),' *Annals of the Royal College of Surgeons of England* 24 no.1 (January 1959): 1-20, https://www.ncbi.nlm.nih.gov/pmc/articles/PMC2413752/ (Accessed February 2022).

4. Dobson, History of the Barbers, 13.

5. Dobson, History of the Barbers, 27.

6. John S. Bolwell, 'The licensing of surgeons by RCS England and its predecessors, *Bulletin of the Royal College of Surgeons of England*. 103, no. 3 (May 2021): E17-24, https://doi.org/10.1308/rcsbull.2021.55 (Accessed January 2022).

7. John R. Guy, 'The Episcopal Licensing of Physicians, Surgeons and Midwives,' *Bulletin of the History of Medicine* 50, no. 4 (Winter 1982): 528-42, THE EPISCOPAL LICENSING OF PHYSICIANS, SURGEONS AND MIDWIVES on JSTOR (Accessed February 2022).

8. Cecil Wall, *The History of the Surgeons' Company 1745-1800* (London: Hutchinson, 1937): 18, https://iiif.wellcomecollection.org/pdf/b29827085 (Accessed December 2021).

9. Bank of England Inflation Calculator https://www.bankofengland.co.uk/monetary-policy/inflation/inflation-calculator (Accessed February 2022)

10. Wall, Surgeons' Company, 37-40.

11. Wall, Surgeons' Company, 49.

12. V. Zachary Cope, *The History of The Royal College of Surgeons of England* (London Blond, 1959): 3-6

13. Sidney Young. *The Annals of the Barber-Surgeons of London* (London: Blades, East & Blades, 1890: 416, https://www.gutenberg.org/files/49011/49011-h/49011-h.htm (Accessed March 2022).

14. Wall, Surgeons' Company, 23.

15. Wall, Surgeons' Company, 28.

16. Wall, Surgeons' Company, 63.

17. Cope, History of the College, 7-15.

18. Cope, History of the College, 55.

19. Cope, History of the College, 16-21.

20. Stephen Paget, *John Hunter: Man of Science and Surgeon* (London: Fisher Unwin, 1897): 244-249, 250-260, https://ia802703.us.archive.org/33/items/johnhuntermanofs00pageuoft/johnhuntermanofs00pageuoft_bw.pdf (Accessed December 2021).

21, Cope, History of the College, 28-31.

22. A. Batty Shaw, 'Benjamin Gooch, eighteenth-century Norfolk surgeon,' *Medical History* 16, no. 1 (January 1972): 42, https://doi.org/10.1017/s0025727300017245 (Accessed February 2022).

23. Cope, History of the College, 39-40.

24. Young, Annals of the Barber-Surgeons, 440

25. Archives of the Royal College of Surgeons of England, '*History of the Coat of Arms,*'https://www.rcseng.ac.uk/about-the-rcs/history-of-the-rcs/coat-of-arms/ (Accessed March 2022)

26. Cope, History of the College, 246-250.

27 *Edward W.* Riley and Laurence Gomme, eds., *Survey of London: Volume 3, St Giles-in-The-Fields, Pt I: Lincoln's Inn Fields* (London: London County Council, 1912): 458, (Footnote 19), https://www.british-history.ac.uk/survey-london/vol3/pt1/pp48-58 (Accessed December 2021).

28. Cope, History of the College, 70-75

29. Archives of the Royal College of Surgeons of England, 'A Brief Architectural History,' Royal College of Surgeons Architectural History (Accessed December 2021)

30. Cope, History of the College, 85

31. The Royal College of Surgeons of England, *Souvenir of the Centenary of the Royal College of Surgeons of England, 1800-1900* (London: Ballantyne Hanson, 1900): 13-16, Souvenir of the Centenary of the Royal College of Surgeons of England, 1800-1900 – Royal College of Surgeons of England - Google Books (Accessed February 2022)

32. Simon Shorvon and Alastair Compston, *Queen Square: A History of the National Hospital and its Institute of Neurology* (Cambridge: Cambridge University Press, (2018): 61.

33. Cope, History of the College, 204-205.

34. Archives of the Royal College of Surgeons of England, (Paper Files: Council 1827 to date), https://aim25.com/cgi-bin/vcdf/detail?coll_id=263&inst_id=9 (Accessed January 2022).

35. Cope, History of the College, 214-221.

36. Alner W. Hall, 'Restoration and Rebuilding of the College; the Nuffield College of Surgical Sciences,' *Annals of the Royal College of Surgeons of England* 17, no. 4 (October 1955): 256-62, https://pubmed.ncbi.nlm.nih.gov/13259416/ (Accessed January 2022).

37. Cyril Long, 'The Institute of Basic Medical Sciences. The first 25 years,' 1951-76, *Annals of the Royal College of Surgeons of England* 59, no. 3 (May 1977): 181-98, https://www.ncbi.nlm.nih.gov/pmc/articles/PMC2491771/ (Accessed December 2021)

38. 'The Nuffield College of Surgical Sciences,' *Annals of the Royal College of Surgeons of England* 20, no. 5 (May 1957): 316-23, https://www.ncbi.nlm.nih.gov/pmc/articles/PMC2413476/pdf/annrcse00325-0051.pdf (Accessed February 2022).

39. Royal College of Surgeons of England, *Plarr's Lives of the Fellows, Alan Parks,* https://livesonline.rcseng.ac.uk/client/en_GB/lives/search/results?qu=Parks&te=ASSET(Accessed December 2021),

40. Timothy M. Lane, 'Plus ça change,' *Annals of the Royal College of Surgeons of England* 102, no. 6 (July 2020): 399-400, https://doi.org/10.1308/rcsann.2020.0144 (Accessed August 2021).

41. Royal College of Surgeons of England, *Plarr's Lives of the Fellows, Raymond Last,* https://livesonline.rcseng.ac.uk/client/en_GB/lives/search/results?qu=Last+Raymond&te=ASSET (Accessed October 2021),

42. Royal College of Surgeons of England, *Plarr's Lives of the Fellows, Rodney Smith,* https://livesonline.rcseng.ac.uk/client/en_GB/lives/search/results?qu=Smith+Rodney&te=ASSET (Accessed October 2021),

43. Royal College of Surgeons of England, *Plarr's Lives of the Fellows, Ronald Johnson-Gilbert,* (Plarr's Lives of the Fellows online only since 2005). https://livesonline.rcseng.ac.uk/client/en_GB/lives/search/results?qu=Johnson-Gilbert&te=ASSET (Accessed October 2021),

44. George Smart, 'The State of British Medicine - 3: The British Postgraduate Medical Federation,' *Journal of the Royal Society of Medicine* 71, no. 6 (March 1978): 167-69, https://doi.org/10.1177/014107687807100303 (Accessed November 2021).

45. 'Flowers Report, London medical education,' *British Medical Journal* 280, no 6215 (March 1980): 731-33, https://www.ncbi.nlm.nih.gov/pmc/articles/PMC1600769/pdf/brmedj00010-0073.pdf (Accessed December 2021).

46. Cope, History of the College, 105.

47. Fahema Begum, *Darwin and Down House,* (2017), Archives of the Royal College of Surgeons of England, https://www.rcseng.ac.uk/library-and-publications/library/blog/darwin-and-down-house/ (Accessed August 2021).

48. The Lord Todd, *Royal Commission on Medical Education* (London: Her Majesty's Stationery Office, Command 3569, Report 1968)

49. Geoffrey Rivett, *From Cradle to Grave: Fifty years of the NHS* (London: King's Fund Publishing, 1997): 15-17, https://archive.kingsfund.org.uk/concern/published_works/000018818 (Accessed June 2021).

50. 'Royal Commission on Medical Education,' *British Medical Journal* 2, no. 5597 (April 1968): 109-11, https://www.bmj.com/content/bmj/2/5597/109.full.pdf (Accessed August 2021).

51. History of Imperial College, Faculty of Medicine, https://www.imperial.ac.uk/medicine/about-us/history/ (Accessed December 2021).

52. Bernard Tomlinson, *Report of the inquiry into London's health service, medical education and research* (London: Her Majesty's Stationery Office, 1968), https://www.sochealth.co.uk/national-health-service/hospitals/tomlinson-report-1992/ ¶110 to ¶143. (Accessed December 2021).

53. Negley Harte, John North and Georgina Brewis, The World of UCL (London: UCL Press, 2018): 59, 70-72, 275-80, https://discovery.ucl.ac.uk/id/eprint/10048692/1/World-of-UCL.pdf (Accessed February 2022)

54. History of King's College, London, https://www.kcl.ac.uk/about/history (Accessed March 2022).

55. History of St. George's, University of London, https://www.sgul.ac.uk/about/who-we-are/history (Accessed October 2021).

56. History of Queen Mary College, London, https://www.qmul.ac.uk/about/history/ (Accessed September 2021).

57. Rivett, Cradle to Grave, 93.

58. Bryan Abel-Smith, *The Hospitals 1800-1948: A Study in Social Administration in England and Wales* (London: Heinemann, 1964): 486-87.

59. Abel-Smith, Hospitals, 480

60. Charles Webster, ed., *Aneurin Bevan on the National Health Service* (Oxford: University of Oxford, Wellcome Unit for the History of Medicine, 1991): 219-22, https://wellcomecollection.org/works/ga2pjwqw (Accessed December 2021)

61. Kenneth C. Calman, *Hospital Doctors: Training for the Future: the Report of the Working Group on Specialist Medical Training* (London: Department of Health, 1993).

62. Mehool Patel, 'Changes to postgraduate medical education in the 21st century,' *Clinical Medicine Journal* 16, no. 4 (August 2016): 311-14, https://www.rcpjournals.org/content/clinmedicine/16/4/311 (Accessed September 2021).

63. Claire Chalmers, Supriya Joshi, Philip Bentley and Nicholas Boyle, 'The Lost Generation: Impact of the 56- hour EWTD on current surgical training,' *Annals of the Royal College of Surgeons of England Supplement* 92, no. 3 (March 2010): 102-6, https://publishing.rcseng.ac.uk/doi/10.1308/147363510X491105 (Accessed October 2021).

64. The Royal College of Surgeons of England, '*Careers in Surgery: Improving Surgical Training,*' (2021), https://www.rcseng.ac.uk/careers-in-surgery/trainees/ (Accessed January 2022).

65. Jon Lund, 'The new General Surgical Curriculum and ISCP,' *Surgery (Oxford)* 38 no. 10 (October 2020): 601-6, https://www.ncbi.nlm.nih.gov/pmc/articles/PMC7462536/ (Accessed December 2021).

66. Naila Dhanani, Oscar Olavarria, Karla Bernardi et al, 'The Evidence Behind Robot-Assisted Abdominopelvic Surgery: A Systematic Review,' *Annals of Internal Medicine* 174, no. 8 (August 2021): 1110-7. https://doi.org/10.7326/M20-7006 (Accessed March 2022).

67. Alan Turing, 'Computing Machinery and Intelligence,' *Mind 59*, no. 236 (October 1950): 433-60, https://doi.org/10.1093/mind/LIX.236.433 (Accessed January 2022).

68. Junaid Bajwa, Usman Munir, Aditya Nori and Bryan Williams, 'Artificial intelligence in healthcare: transforming the practice of medicine,' *Future Healthcare Journal 8*, no. 2 (July 2021): E188-94, https://doi.org/10.7861/fhj.2021-0095 (Accessed January 2022).

69. Harold Luft, John Bunker and Alain Enthoven, 'Should operations be regionalized? The empirical relation between surgical volume and mortality,' *The New England Journal of Medicine* 301, no. 25 (December 1979): 1364-69, https://doi.org/10.1056/NEJM197912203012503 (Accessed February 2022).

70. Hartwig Bauer, Kim Honselmann and Andrew Warshaw, 'Minimum Volume Standards in Surgery - Are We There Yet?' *Visceral Medicine* 33, no. 2 (April 2017): 106-16, https://doi.org/10.1159/000456041 (Accessed December 2021).

71. NHS England, 'The NHS Long Term Plan,' London: NHS, (2019), https://www.england.nhs.uk/commissioning/spec-services/ (Accessed December 2021).

72. NHS England, 'The NHS Long Term Plan,' London: NHS, (2019), 56-63, https://www.longtermplan.nhs.uk/wp-content/uploads/2019/08/nhs-long-term-plan-version-1.2.pdf (Accessed December 2021).

73. Frank Heynick, 'The original "magic bullet" is 100 years old,' British Journal of Psychiatry 195, no. 5 (November 2009): 456, https://doi.org/10.1192/bjp.195.5.456 (Accessed December 2021).

74. Howard Markel, 'The ugly truth behind the discovery of DNA,' The Washington Post, 13 September 2021, https://www.washingtonpost.com/outlook/2021/09/13/ugly-truth-behind-discovery-dna/ (Accessed February 2022).

75. Howard Markel, The Secret of Life: Rosalind Franklin, James Watson, Francis Crick, and the Discovery of DNA's Double Helix (New York: Norton, 2021).

76. Ian Donald, John MacVicar and Thomas Brown, 'Investigation of abdominal masses by pulsed ultrasound,' The Lancet 271 no. 7032 (June 1958):1188-95, https://doi.org/10.1016/S0140-6736(58) 91905-6 (Accessed February 2022).

77. Avedis Donabedian, Explorations in Quality Assessment and Monitoring. Vol I. The definition of quality and approaches to its assessment, 1980; Vol II. The criteria and standards of quality, 1982; Vol III. The methods and findings of quality assessment and monitoring: an illustrated analysis (Ann Arbor: Health Administration Press, 1985).

78. Archibald L. Cochrane, Effectiveness and Efficiency: Random Reflections on Health Services (The Rock Carling Fellowship 1971) (London: Nuffield Provincial Hospitals Trust, 1972).

79. Stuart Weir and David Beetham, Political Power and Democratic Control in Britain: The Democratic Audit of the United Kingdom (London: Routledge, 1999), 224.

80. Rahee Mapara, Clara Munro, Mobolaji Ajekigbe and Greta McLachlan, eds. 'Sexism, racism and homophobia at the Royal College of Surgeons of England.' *British Medical Journal* 373; no. 998 (20 April 2021). doi: https://doi.org/10.1136/bmj.n998 (Accessed March 2022).

81. Royal College of Surgeons of England, *Diversity, Equity and Inclusion Action Plan,* (London: RCS England, 2021), https://www.rcseng.ac.uk/about-the-rcs/about-our-mission/diversity/action-plan/#Plan (Accessed February 2022)

82. Zulekha Nathoo. *Why ineffective diversity training won't go away* (London: BBC WorkLife, 14 June 2021), https://www.bbc.com/worklife/article/20210614-why-ineffective-diversity-training-wont-go-away (Accessed February 2022)

Ingram Content Group UK Ltd.
Milton Keynes UK
UKHW021049120323
418359UK00011B/133